Married Couples
Thou Shalt Have Great Sex

Married Couples
Thou Shalt Have Great Sex

Undressing Issues and Exposing Topics That Inhibit Sensual Sexual Pleasure (Eden)

Helping Married Couples "KNOW" each other Intimately

T. Charles Brantley M. Div

**Outskirts Press, Inc.
Denver, Colorado**

The opinions expressed in this manuscript are solely the opinions of the author and do not represent the opinions or thoughts of the publisher. The author has represented and warranted full ownership and/or legal right to publish all the materials in this book.

Married Couples: Thou Shalt Have Great Sex
Undressing Issues and Exposing Topics That Inhibit Sexual Pleasure (Eden)
All Rights Reserved.
Copyright © 2009 T. Charles Brantley
v3.0

This book may not be reproduced, transmitted, or stored in whole or in part by any means, including graphic, electronic, or mechanical without the express written consent of the publisher except in the case of brief quotations embodied in critical articles and reviews.

Outskirts Press, Inc.
http://www.outskirtspress.com

ISBN: 978-1-4327-4118-1

Outskirts Press and the "OP" logo are trademarks belonging to Outskirts Press, Inc.

PRINTED IN THE UNITED STATES OF AMERICA

Song of Solomon 4

[3] Your lips are like a scarlet ribbon;
your mouth is lovely.
Your temples behind your veil
are like the halves of a pomegranate.

[4] Your neck is like the tower of David,
built with courses of stone;
on it hang a thousand shields,
all of them shields of warriors.

[5] Your breasts are like two fawns,
like twin fawns of a gazelle
that browse among the lilies.

<u>Today's New International Version</u>. Zondervan, 2005.

Table of Contents

Introduction 3
Agape, Philia, & Eros 11
Spiritual and Sensual 19
Balance the Spiritual and the Sexual 27
The Golden Rule 39
60/40 Rule 45
FORGIVENESS 53
Home First; Ministry Second 57
If He Stops, What Will You Do, Wives? 65
Seeds of Divorce 75
Stimulus Package: Sex as a Tool—Not as a Weapon ... 81
Have an Affair with Your Spouse 89
Power of Mutual Submission 113
Remove the Chastity Belt 119
Problems with Sex 127
Fears of Sex 135
The Matrix 145
Sarah's Pleasure 151
Femme Fatale 159
Tori Amos: The Voice of a Generation 177
Victorian Morality 187
Church Attitudes on Sex from Antiquity 197
Celibacy 205
Knew (Biblical Word for Sex) 209
SEX on the Brain: Releasing Hormones 221
Lingerie and Sexy Underwear 235
Argentine Lake Duck (Size Can Scare You) 241
Your Member Has an Expiration Date 247
IT IS NOT NASTY 255
Conclusion 265

INTRODUCTION

Introduction

In my spiritual travels, I have seen many people carry a banner of ethics of their own creation instead of the Lord's. Many times our individual Christian ethical standards go beyond God's commandments. In some circumstances, we take OUR Word to a higher level to outshine Christ the Redeemer. We cannot reside under a banner of legalism to save ourselves. We must instead reside under the banner of grace. Not to abuse grace, but to appreciate what God did through the life, death, resurrection, and ascension of Jesus, the Christ.

We read and hear that the divorce rate is the same (or even higher) in the Christian population as it is in the secular world. Some of us may just skip over this fact, but such words give me pause and make me want to ponder this point. If we Christians have the answers, and if we know how to classify sin, why are we failing at something that God instituted? God hates divorce. Jesus only gave one reason for it in 5 Matthew, but it seems many of us are not listening to Him. According to the *Christian Post Reporter*'s Audrey Barrick,

After months of revived debate over divorce and its increasing acceptance among Americans, a new study affirmed born again Christians are just as likely as the average American couple to divorce.

The Barna Group found in its latest study that born again Christians who are not evangelical were indistinguishable from the national average on the matter of divorce with 33 percent having married and divorced at least once. Among all born again Christians, which includes evangelicals, the divorce figure is 32 percent, which is statistically identical to the 33 percent figure among non-born again adults, the research group noted. (*Christian Post Reporter*, **Apr 04 2008)**[1]

I must confess that marriage is no walk in the park. It is a road paved with difficulties. However, with Christ, ALL things are possible. It seems that Christians just apply their power to battles against Satan and do not apply that power to their marriages. I submit that the biggest problems come from inside the home rather than outside the home. If we can learn to battle and win our wars at home, we will have more victories outside the home.

Let us take this further. When you have trouble at home, you cannot relax because you have a battle in your own dwelling. Yet, when the home front is free from issues and problems, you have a place of rest from the works of the enemy. Over time, a married couple can, without thinking, drift away from each other; that is the time when you must pull out the scriptures and combat this trial of the enemy within your own residence.

When you deal with marriage, do so not just through a spiritual microscope; you must also use what I call 'a flesh-magnification glass.' **To use 'a flesh-magnification glass' is to respect the flesh and not ignore it. As married couples wielding this glass, you respect the need for sexual relationships without condemnation.** This is difficult for many Christians to swallow, especially those of the Holiness persuasion, but we are not yet in our heavenly suits: we still have to deal with the flesh. The flesh is not going anywhere. In fact, you and I will deal with this flesh until Jesus the Christ comes back again.

Jesus did pray in the book of John that we would not be taken out of the world but that we would be kept in the world (John 17:11). I believe that the reason why divorce occurs in the body of Christ is because people do not understand that marriage must be waged both inside and outside of the bedroom. In fact, a couple's sex and intimacy must be as much a priority in their lives as reading the Bible and attending church. Yet hindrances arise to obstruct the road to successful intimacy. In *Rekindling Desire*, Barry & Emily McCarthy say,

"Making the psychological, relational and situational changes that are necessary to enjoy pleasure, arousal and orgasm is doable, but not simple. Sometimes the couple loses motivation and focus. The longer the dysfunction exists, the more likely it will result in inhibited sexual desire."(McCarty 2003)[2]

So, couples, you have to fight to keep sex alive. Moreover, Christians, I am telling you, the answer is not "Just pray," it's get into bed and "Just do it!" Keep reading, and we will cover more specifics on that aspect later in this book. Those of the ascetic bent want to crucify the flesh. Yes, scripture speaks of this, but when you are married, there exists a line of demarcation (not having sex) that you must not cross.

Although most Protestants do not observe celibacy, many married Christians practice celibacy emotionally and spiritually for various reasons. This is not the will of God. Hence, this book is written to help couples reconcile what the Bible says and translate that into their homes and especially their bedrooms. Let us understand first and foremost: God wants those of us who have walked down the aisle to be happily married. Because of this, we need to understand that a happy marriage in a Christian home also means happiness in the bedroom.

Many Christians have the spiritual side down pat. Oh yes, they know how to love God, give alms, and even speak in tongues. However, when it comes to the woman or man they married, well, now, that is another story. We need to re-write that story to save couples from themselves. Yes, you need to know God (spiritually), but you also need to know your spouse (sensually). Those two words—sensual and spiritual—should be part of our marriage vocabulary. We cannot ignore this, and those who do might find themselves walking down the aisle to divorce.

This book will not pull any punches. I will say whatever it takes to get you and your spouse into a happy sexual partnership. We cannot love God and want to save the world and not use that same power to save our own marriages. We cannot say we love God and not love our brothers, sisters, and especially, our spouse. We see this written in 1 John 3. Well, my brother and sister, that love must first be shared in the family before it's shared in the world. What good is it to save the world while your family goes to hell physically and emotionally?

One solution for couples is to re-learn the love of God and each other. Yet, many Christian couples focus on their

Agape love and not their love of Eros. (I will discuss these forms of love in the next section). Basically, Agape love represents the foundation, but couples cannot ignore the Eros love that wells up within them. When you ignore your God-given desires, you only hurt yourself and, ultimately, your sexual relationship with your spouse.

I do not mean to sound crude, but going to the bathroom is a natural human function. We have all experienced holding it in longer than we wanted. Well, when Christian couples do not address their sexual needs—and when I say sexual needs I mean having orgasms—they only create problems within their marriage.

I understand how couples get to this point, and we will walk through this process; the key, though, is working our way out of this bubble that denies married Christian couples what the Lord has designed. In the book of Genesis, God looked down at what He had created and called everything good, and, yes, that included sex. Logically, when you let God fill all the blank spaces in your life, your spouse will be the frosting on the cake.

There is no way that your spouse knows all the areas that are needed to satisfy you. Your spouse is not your creator. Your spouse's first job is to provide companionship and ensure that you are not alone. We forget that before woman, God was in company with man. God walked and talked with man. Yet, God knew that man needed sex. Hence, God created woman. Everything that man needed came from God. Man had no wants or desires, yet when it came to his loins, God recognized a need, backed up, and created woman.

This shows us that God approves of sex because He created it; He recognized man's need to satisfy his overwhelming desires. If God wanted man to be celibate or alone, there would have been no need for woman. If God hated sex, he would have left man as he was, but he knew that man needed sex. Since God created sex, sex must be good. If God wanted man to refrain from sexual activity, he would have not created woman. If God made woman just so Adam had someone to chat with, then God would not have given woman a vagina and man a penis. Since He created both, sex is good. We all must face this fact. God created it, and sex is good.

We have been told through the ages to deny the flesh, but in so doing, we have hindered many Christian married couples from enjoying the passion and pleasure that was made by the hand of God. Too many married couples talk about everything else but what pleases them in bed and what "menu" they want for that night. Get over it Christian couples, the sex is there. So what will you do with it? I hope that this book will encourage husbands and wives to investigate this great gift from God.

References
1. Barrick, Audrey. Study: Christian divorce rate identical to national average. 2008. Christian Post-Reporter, Apr 04 2008.<http://www.christianpost.com/Society/Polls_reports/2008/04/study-christian-divorce-rate-identical-to-national-average-04/index.html>
2. McCarthy, Barry W. & McCarthy, Emily J. Rekindling desire: A step-by-step program to help low-sex and no-sex marriages. New York, Routledge. (2003).

AGAPE, PHILIA, & EROS

Agape, Philia, & Eros

Humans experience three types of love. *Agape* love refers to love one gives without reciprocity, i.e., from the kindness of one's heart. *Philia* is more of a friendship type of love. *Eros* reflects sexual drive (libido) and feelings. Traditionally, the church has correctly focused on Agape and Philia love. However, for a married couple, there are times to attend to Eros or sexual drive. Agape love is accomplished with God's help. Our human nature is to give love and get it back. Yet when it comes to God, He gives without any type of reciprocity. His son, Jesus the Christ, proved this. He gave us Christ when we deserved death and damnation. Scripture said while we were yet sinners, Christ died for our sins. He gave love without looking for any return.

I have found that the amount of love a spouse gives to his or her spouse does not necessarily equal the love returned, as in perfect reciprocity. Many times, when a husband or a wife gives love, the partner in the relationship will not experience the same feelings of happiness. For this reason, a spouse must first get this love from God and then from the spouse. God's love is never ending—it will never run out, but our love does. Women tend to focus on Philia, but men focus on the Eros.

However, men, when Eros love between you and wife is not working, then work on Philia or Agape love. Wives, when Agape or Philia is not working, work on the Eros. Instead of cursing the definition of love, try to focus on the type of love that is working. Please understand that marriage is complex. If it were not complex, the divorce rate would not be so high. By breaking down marriage, you can identify what areas need growth and what areas need fixing.

This is why couples cannot just focus on Philia without Eros. They cannot focus on Eros without Philia. The three points must work in harmony. In my mind, the diagram goes like this: Both partners must go to God for Agape love—the type of love that does not look for reciprocity. Again, couples, go together to God for this. When we put His Agape love in place, we will be able to love one another in holy matrimony.

Too many couples have Agape love at the altar, but after the marriage ceremony, they leave it there. By accepting and exercising the perfect example of love, couples can work on Eros love with each other. **Again, the reason why couples cannot love is that they have not learned from the greatest LOVER, GOD.** Yes, God is the greatest lover because He gave when we did not deserve His love. Again, this is the purest form of love. Just as God loves and forgives those who ask, once we love and forgive again, we are on the road to save our marriages and ourselves.

You cannot say you have love and not recognize and learn from the One who loves us the most. Following His loving example, we can have Philia and Eros with our spouses. And do not forget, on those occasions when your wife or husband disappoints you, you always have Agape love to turn to: That is a powerful application. We cannot go to man or woman for the relief of pain. God is the true healer.

When distance develops between them and couples do not experience or seek out Agape love, they have no way of handling the pain. Yet the opposite is true for couples that have surrounded themselves with the love of the Lord. I am not saying God's love is supplemental; God's love is essential to building the foundation for all other types of love to flourish. Therefore, when you have the foundation installed and know in your heart all three types of love, only then you can embrace Eros love without fear of failure. You cannot fail because you have the power of God's love as your foundation.

Remember that neither Philia nor Eros can be the foundation of a marriage. Only Agape can be the foundation of a marriage. Yet Agape love opens the door to physical (sexual) issues. When you go to the extremes, some couples have a spiritual answer for physical issues. I consider them super-deep people who need to get a grip on the real issues facing them. Too much of anything is not good. When we look at the broad landscape of Christians, we sometimes see people who hide behind their super-spiritual mindsets to avoid dealing with marriage issues. As Tim Alan Gardner and Stanley Scott write in *Sacred Sex* (2002),"It's time for Christians to bring the idea of sex and holiness together."[1]

I believe in the power of prayer and Bible study. Yet, once we get the revelations from the Lord, we must put them into action. Just as the Bible's Sarah and Abraham had to put their faith into action (to produce Isaac), so do all married couples. It is time for married couples to hook up. I am not just talking about sex, but all avenues of marriage.

When an individual experiences troubling issues in marriage, he or she must first seek the Lord. However, after seeking the Lord, that person must apply to the marriage what was learned from the Lord. This is the missing link for Christian couples today. It is either feast or famine. Either they have too much God or they have too much Eros. Within a loving couple, the key word is **balance**.

Before we conclude this chapter, couples should be honest. Before getting married, you may have failed to know all three forms of love. It is a hard thing to learn something when you are an adult. I have heard people say that because they never learned how to swim, they are afraid of water. Because their parents never gave them the gift of learning to swim, they have lost the enjoyment of what surrounds over three-quarters of the earth.

Well, the same holds true in marriages everyday. Because some adults never learned the three forms of love in action, they find it nearly impossible to swim in this new element. In addition, because they never learned it as a child, they are unable to offer their spouse what the spouse needs. If you never saw love in your home, unless God performs a miracle, you will always be at the short end of the stick. **This is a powerful statement because so many homes are broken, and kids learn to fight instead of to love. Kids learn how to get divorced instead of how to stay together.**

Given these histories, these kids are now adults in their own marriages, and, because the three types of love have not been properly modeled, they are now at a disadvantage with their spouse. They are unsure of what to do and how to do it. Due to the lack of this knowledge, instead of floating on love, they drown. Couples must know they are together in the vessel of love, and they must relearn love.

If they do not learn, they can easily find themselves in a sexless marriage. According to "Dealing with a Sexless Marriage," by Juju Chang and Cole Kazdin,

"Sex may be on television, in the theaters and advertising, but it's not in the homes of 20 million American couples that are in sexless marriages. Once a taboo topic, sexless marriages are getting more attention, in part because so many couples are complaining about the lack of sexual activity in their unions, according to one gynecologist. "

"It's an epidemic… In a sexless marriage, couples only are sexually intimate 10 or fewer times a year."[2]

Instead of suffering, Christian couples can teach one another not only Agape love but also Eros love. This is the main advantage that couples have: they can now teach one another how to really love. This is when you get out the Bible and other books on marriage and learn or relearn how to love one another. Some couples take this limitation, make it into a disadvantage, and turn their marriages into loveless situations. It should be the other way around. Learn to make this an advantage. Learn to do things differently together. When you learn together, you define together.

This will not be an overnight or quick fix. It may take a lifetime to come up with answers for these issues. You have to constantly redefine and rethink, and, over time, things will change. For example, as you grow older, the Eros may not be there, as you so desire. Meaning there may be times when one spouse may want to have sex but the other wants to cuddle. This is where compromise comes into play.

Saints of the highest God, we cannot ignore that there

are issues in the body of Christ when it comes to marriage, but you must fight on! I know it is going to be tough and difficult at times but you must fight to learn ALL the parts of love. Yes, that includes the sensual part.

As a three-legged stool cannot stand on two legs, the same is true of a marriage. If just two legs are present, the stool will fall. If one of the three is short, the stool will teeter uncomfortably. This is what I say to couples. Make sure the stool works. You must have all three types of love in your marriage. Oh, yes, when you are really in tune with yourself and God and spouse, you will reach the peak of all types of love.

However, such things are rare because so much junk can get in your way that can and will stop couples from their goal of mutual love. Yet, through God's grace, you can undo the pain of the past and reach for your future, and then you will see a great harvest within your marriage.

References
1. Gardner, Tim Alan, & Stanley, Scott. <u>Sacred sex: A spiritual celebration of oneness in marriage</u>. Colorado Springs, CO: WaterBrook Press, 2002
2. Chang, Juju, & Kazdin, Cole. <u>Dealing with a sexless marriage: Scheduling sex, being realistic may help improve your intimacy with your partner.</u> 2009. ABC NEWS. Feb. 16, 2009 <http://abcnews.go.com/GMA/OnCall/story?id=6884255&page=1>

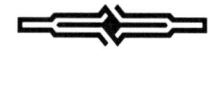

SPIRITUAL AND SENSUAL

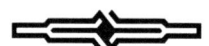

Spiritual and Sensual

The word *sensual* relates to the senses (hearing, sight, smell, touch, taste, and equilibrium). You can include hunger as part of this group as well. When we were born, we were given BOTH spiritual and sensual NEEDS. Both come from God. Because of this, we have to address both issues as we grow in grace.

Many have tried to kill the flesh (the sensual side). Nevertheless, if we are honest with ourselves, we know the flesh rises again. The revelation that I have received is about learning to control and balance these senses. You may not agree, but people can become strict legalists to the point that they do not address their physical issues. I know this sentiment may not be popular, but I see overweight Christian giants who love the Lord but hate their own bodies; we need to learn to love our bodies.

Let me say quickly, yes, we are to crucify the flesh yet only to a certain extent. If we took this scripture literally, then we would all commit suicide because crucifying the flesh would include hunger and going to the bathroom. Again, I emphasize controlling the flesh under the banner of God's power and might. How can you love God and destroy his creation? Your body is God's creation and all the things within it.

We must understand that not only does God want us to love Him, but also He wants us to enjoy our senses in the proper environment. In essence, we cannot continue to love God and hate what He put in place. You cannot hate the one and love the other. Christian couples, we cannot be so in love with the Bible that we do not submit and love one another.

Yes, even in response to bedroom needs. Christian couples can find themselves confused on this point because, as singles they were taught, correctly, to abstain from fornication. Yet, when they marry, the switch is not complete, and they continue withholding sex after marriage. This is not correct. If couples continue to deny each other comfort, divorce may result.

Stephen Sims writes in *Spice up Your Marriage* (2008), "The benefits of spicing up your marriage are profound. Virtually every area of my life has improved by investing in my committed relationship. The promise of a vastly improved life experience for both of us completes a compelling argument."[1] This is why I help couples start the balancing act of the spiritual and sensual. A Christian couple cannot fast throughout the relationship. In fact, couples need to look at sex as a part of the system. If the system is not working in one area, then you will have a problem in another. Your senses are all connected. If one part is denied and suffocates, the other parts suffer.

For example, when blood stops flowing to any of our extremities, atrophy or a kind of sleep, happens to that area. In addition, it hurts a lot to get the blood flowing again. Well, I am trying to say that when you are flowing, so to speak, in one area of your marriage (spiritual) and not in another area (sexual), you will hurt the body or marriage as a whole. Christian couples, God has given us a balm called sex.

When this area of your married life is not fulfilled, or when you try to apply a spiritual solution, you will have problems down the road. God has given us the tools, but it is up to us to use the tools. In addition, please do not forget that if your tool goes unused, it will gather cobwebs and rust. Well, Christian couples, dust off the cobwebs and get busy. I am not telling you to become a sex addict. Balance is the word for today. Focusing totally on sex to the point that you forget the spiritual side creates dangers as well. As in everything, you cannot overcompensate.

You must not have a caught-up spirit. You must just take it one day at a time and learn to put into place what God has already given to couples. Sex is not the priority here. God is the priority. He is the foundation of our faith and life. Paul said that we live, move, and have our being by God. **However, we still have this flesh and it has needs that require tending.**

For married couples, the large elephant in the bedroom is called sex. Couples who ignore it will find themselves in bad situations. This occurs because the body and mind say: let us have sex after marriage. In addition, when you continue to ignore a natural human need, you hinder the marriage. Yes, you have God, but you do not have companionship—even though you took the marriage vows. This is why Christian couples must balance spirit and sex. One goes with the other. You cannot do it one-sidedly.

In a way, God has defined the spiritual side for us through His Word, but the sexual side is defined between each couple. When I say defined, I mean they discuss what areas they will and will not enter, within their marriage. Marriage is still defined between one man and one woman. Each couple has different needs, wants, and desires.

When we are single, God should be the priority. Yet after marriage, the spouse becomes just as important. One cannot use God in a sexual situation. Your spouse fulfills sexual roles within your life. There is no spiritual solution to this. When I say spiritual, I mean you cannot pray away your sexual appetite in the marriage relationship. Couples must come together, reconcile any issues, and move on to the next level of love and understanding.

Before going further, let me say, you cannot worship God to the point that your spouse becomes envious. Understand my point. If within a marriage one spouse worships God in full glory without abandon and yet enters the marriage bedroom coldly and unwillingly, something is terribly wrong. If you can worship God freely and without regard, you can love your spouse in the same manner.

All couples have issues, and all couples must work through them to get to the other side. Worshiping God is a form of intimacy, and a problem arises if one spouse can love God and not the other spouse. I know terrible things can get in the way, like adultery and lying. Yet if those accounts are resolved and each couple lives and breathes in the truth, there should be no problem in sharing love with each other.

I wrote this book to help couples cross the bridge together as it relates to being spiritual and sensual with one another. At times, spouses may have to help each other cross the bridge on spiritual matters and sexual things. The two must work together. I know this may be deep, but God requires such actions. He told husbands to love their wives as Christ loves the church. This is a commandment from God.

Hence, I must not just love God. I must love my wife. I must give my wife what is due to her to the maximum. Nothing should be held back or lacking. In fact, the dedication that I show to my spouse should resemble the dedication I show to God. Do not get me wrong. God is Number One. Yet, after God, my love for my spouse comes in a close second place.

When you love your spouse, you love God. When you hate your spouse, you hate God. To deny an aspect of marriage, including sex, is to deny the true and living God. He gave marriage as a gift. The spiritual one gave us a sensual gift. To deny the gift is to deny the One who gave the gift. This is why we must walk together on spiritual and sensual paths when we marry. Both aspects are important. When one suffers, the whole body follows.

The constant battle is to find the right mix between spiritual and sensual. This is an ongoing balance between husband and wife. It is ongoing because things always change in a relationship. As Ecclesiastes 3 reminds us, there are times of love and times of hate. The same applies toward couples.

This is why in marriage you cannot forget one and focus on the other. You cannot just say, "I will be spiritual and forget the sensual part of a marriage." I have seen this happen on many occasions, when one spouse gets frustrated with the other; they turned off the sensual, and only focused on the spiritual. Such reactions only lead to trouble. You must maintain both paths all the time.

If you do not, you will be blindsided by the issue that has gone lacking. Whatever you do not feed (spiritually, emotionally, or sexually) will become a problem later on in life. If you continue to feed the spiritual and starve the sensual, you will have trouble. Again, I speak of feeding the sensual side as it relates to marriage. The one needs the other to help the marriage survive. **Yes, God is the foundation, but sex and communication make up the framework of the foundation.**

However, without a building, the foundation will just simply erode. Marriage is about taking God at your wedding, into your marriage, and, especially, into your bedroom. Once you have God in the marriage, you need to build on that foundation. Why do couples often break up after the children leave the house? There is no building on top of the foundation. Speaking from a non-spiritual aspect, communication is the foundation, but sensuality is the framework that keeps marriages together.

Reference
1. Simes, Stephen. <u>Spice up your Marriage: In search of fun, commitment and passion</u>. iDevelop, Ltd.2008

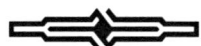

BALANCE THE SPIRITUAL AND THE SEXUAL

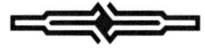

Balance the Spiritual and the Sexual

This is the essence of this book: balance. How can I balance my human desire for sex and my love for God? For the unmarried among us, the answer is easy, but fulfilling it is hard. Singles are not supposed to have sex; not only because of God's law, but also the consequences are too difficult to justify. One sex act can cause a baby, disease, or heartbreak—and we see why God said no. However, for the married couple, God answered that challenging question when He told Adam and Eve to be fruitful and multiply.

How can I insure that I do not neglect one or the other—the sexual and the spiritual? The best way to answer this question is to understand that good married sex comes from God and is within God. When you have great sex with your spouse, you are pleasing God. When you keep God in first-place and take care of the needs of your spousal issues, I guarantee the two will not collide.

Due to our Victorian inheritance and upbringings, in

some cases, people often think that the spiritual and the sexual cannot coexist. They say, "If you love married sex, you are wrong. Love God and ignore married sex, and you are right." I say <u>not so</u> to both. You must understand that sex is a part of the marriage. When you do not have great sex, you hurt the marriage. <u>By saying "No" to great sex, you say "No" to your marriage</u>. Yes, I said it, and I believe it.

SEX is part of the marriage. The Victorian Age left the world with repressed attitudes toward sex, even implying that sex is only for procreation. It also implied that if a wife had sexual pleasure with her husband, she was a bad or loose woman. If a wife has sex with procreation in mind, then all is well in society. In essence, the husband has all the pleasure and the wife has all the work. Such is not fair and does not reflect the will of God in a marriage.

Countless religions have tried to separate the spiritual from sexual pleasure within the married bedroom. For example, one such sect in the first century, Montanism held that the ascetic mind frame of strict moral rules should carry even into the bedroom for married couples. In some households, this same spirit lingers today. People, and this includes some so-called spiritual leaders, try to take people to severe lengths that God has not condoned.

In fact, the New Testament even talks about men who would not allow people to marry at all (1 Timothy 4:3). I believe this mind frame sprang from a preacher who could not bless his wife with an orgasm. Instead of learning to please his wife, he tells others not to have the experience that God has given to all married couples. One thing leads to the next, and before we know it, others are preaching celibacy.

Christians understand <u>bene</u>diction, but according to Dr.

R. C. Sproul, God observed a <u>mal</u>ediction when He saw Adam by himself.[1] Man needed companionship and a part of that companionship included man and woman having great sex. Let me first say, I understand that as Christians, our first job is our relationship with God, but after the Lord, when we are married, we have a spouse to please. I do not understand where one spouse gets off saying, "Yes," to the spirit but "No," to the sensual needs of his or her spouse.

God made man to worship Him, but He also gave man Eve, because man was alone. Man was not alone, because God was there. His spirit needed nothing else in the presence of God. However, when it came to the human touch, man missed something: Adam was missing a mate.

He was missing a woman. Genesis 2:18 says, "And the Lord God said, it is not good that the man should be alone; I will make him a help meet for him." The first thing that gets my attention here is that the Lord God saw that man was not made to be alone. God and Adam saw how the animals had mates after their own kind, but man did not have any companion or procreation abilities after his kind. It is amazing that the Lord God said this.

Now, my point is, if the Lord God saw that is was not good for man to be alone, why then do so-called men of God deny this observation of the Lord God? The Lord is Jehovah or the self-existent One—the official name of the Jewish and Christian God. The Self-Existent One saw Adam alone. The point here is that the God of the universe saw a problem with man's being alone. The problem needed to be fixed.

This is why this book is important: because some people have been single for a long time, they have not crossed over into the married bedroom. Once they jump into the bedroom, they have no clue what to do. **I do understand that when you are single, you are with God alone, but once you marry, your mind frame has to change to a different format. That format pleases both the spiritual and the sensual parts.**

In the midst of the beautiful Garden of Eden, man missed something. Men, this is the point. If you are married, you should not be alone in your bedroom. Therefore, since I have established that God does not want us to be alone, that we as married men and women must learn to balance the spiritual (our walk with God) and the sensual (with our mates satisfied in and out of the bedroom).

We cannot excuse behavior that on one hand goes absolutely crazy for God and worship, but on the other hand—when it comes to being with a spouse sexually—does not follow through to fulfillment with excitement and joy. Genesis 2:18 squarely tells us this was not the idea. This idea—man and woman in loving sensual relations—came from God alone.

Man did not walk up to God and tug on His robe and say, "Hey, God, I think you missed something." God alone saw the plight of man and made a change. He understood that all the beasts of the field had companions except for man.

Therefore, if God said, "Let's get this sensual thing of companionship and love going," what is wrong with those who indulge in the act who are married? Absolutely nothing. Since God instituted marriage, He's the one who can change the rules. Last I read the rules have not changed. Therefore, since the rules have not changed, why do we want to change the rules? When I speak of changing the rules, I speak in part to those spiritual leaders who deny or ignore the power of companionship and sensual love between husband and wife.

Yes, some men and women know how to talk to God, but they cannot talk to their spouse. Let me first say, no man is an expert in talking to his wife, yet he should attempt the task. Yet, some men are so holy that they save their language for God and never take the time to talk to their spouses. This ought not to be. If God said, "Let there be marriage," then who am I to turn the married couple's bedroom into a monk's cell? No, these things ought not to be. As important as our spiritual well-being is, so is the sensual well-being of husband and wife.

The Unger Bible notes that God was not happy with a sexless or unisexual race. Again, if God was not happy, neither should Christians be who are married but having no sex in their bedrooms. The pressure not to enjoy married sex comes not only from unknowledgeable preachers, but also sometimes from singles who have been hurt and who influence unhappily married friends. If celibacy is your thing, then it is your thing. But do not decide to go celibate after you are married.

Everyday, in a church somewhere, the guilt trip is laid on married couples to love only God (and not their spouses in the sexual way). You may ask why I am so persistent in talking about sensual marriage relationship. Simple. For ages, we had chastity and not enough teaching about sensual love between husband and wife. In fact, many still linger in the twilight zone and do not talk of or even acknowledge the sensual side of marriage.

However, if God said that man is good, then every aspect of him is good. That includes the sexual part. Through the ages, people have tried to demonize the flesh. For example, Docetism purported that Christ was only spirit, and the flesh only *appeared* real. This belief arose because people were trying to separate flesh from spirit. The same spirit lingers with us today. But know this: we cannot demonize the flesh without demonizing the plan of God as it relates to married sex. The flesh is not wrong in and of itself. It is only wrong in the wrong application. In the single life, sex is wrong. In marriage, sex is right.

People of antiquity acknowledged the good of the spirit, but, on the other hand, they demonized the flesh. Plato and Aristotle tried to tackle the question of *ontology* or the nature of being. One separated it, while the other tried to mutate it. The key again is: antiquity demonized the flesh. That same spirit of Docetism—of hating the flesh—lives on within those who debate the flesh to the point that they deny the sensual side of marriage. Get over this: such should not be the "soup-of-the-day."

Instead, we find the soup-of-the-day for married couples in Genesis 1:28: "Be fruitful, multiply and replenish the earth." We cannot get away from this first order given to man. In addition, we cannot deny that while procreation is going on, there is also pleasure going on along with the act. In fact, if there were no pleasure involved, wives would not want to have sex. Therefore, God in His wisdom gave us pleasure to go along with the act. In addition, if procreation is not the goal, the pleasure is still there.

What some religious folks have tried to do is take the pleasure out of sex. You cannot do the act and separate the emotional and physical. Through ungodly teaching in some circles, false teachers have created this separation—a separation that was not intended by God. Say with me, "Pleasure and sex go together." They are not separated. God did not separate the two, so why should we? If a couple is married, such separation of sex and pleasure should not take place.

When married couples have sex, and they do it to honor their commitment to God, they glorify him. They can be both spiritual and sensual—spiritual in the sense that they love God <u>and</u> sensual in how they reach other. Yet, if a couple commits adultery, they do not glorify what God has ordained.

In continuing to think about sex and pleasure, we turn to data from Dr. Yvonne K. Fulbright[2], who says having (married) sex is healthier than going to the gym and sweating things out. According to a Fox News story, the benefits of sex include the following added bonuses:

1. Weight loss: We burn 200 to 300 calories in 30 minutes. (Minute Men need to improve by 29 minutes!)
2. Pain management: During sexual arousal and orgasm, we release beneficial endorphins and corticosteroids that ease aches and pains. This may explain why so many Christian couples (who refrain from sex) look mean and unhappy. They have spiritual management, but no sensual-pain management. I am not speaking heresy. I am only saying that God has given married couples something besides His Word to bring us comfort. It goes beyond "The Lord is my shepherd." If you are married, it's "I am going to lie down in your green pastures (with my spouse)."
3. Stress release, sleep enhancement, and mood lifting: Sexual arousal increases our levels of Oxytocin and simulates feelings of warmth and relaxation, helping our ability to sleep, and elevating our emotions.

4. Immune booster: Sex helps us fight off colds and flu. Is it possible that the reason why we have an increase in prescriptions and doctor visits is that married couples are not pleasing each other in the bedroom? Yes, we go to church, give praise, and worship, but we must not forget 1 Corinthians 7:5: "Defraud ye not one the other, except [it be] with consent for a time, that ye may give yourselves to fasting and prayer; and come together again, that Satan tempt you not for your incontinency."
5. Improved heart health: We get a cardiovascular workout while making love. (It also lowers cholesterol and heart attacks.) Many men do not understand, for example, that a weak erection signals that blood is not flowing to the penis. In addition, erections occur because the heart pumps blood to the penis. If, however, the blood does flow to the penis, then the male can attend to the needs of his wife. In fact, when a male cannot become erect, it is his heart telling him something is wrong. In the ancient world, people did not have the luxury of today's medicine, but they had the penis as a guide to the strength of the heart.
6. A better, younger-looking you: Sex releases DHEA (dehydroepiandrostone)—the youth-producing hormone. The more you do the more you produce. (Plastic surgeons would go out of business!)
7. Reduced risk of breast cancer in women and prostate cancer in men.

I will elaborate on the physical attributes of sex in another part of this book.

In short, God has given us sex and sexual pleasure—

sex did not come from *Playboy* or *Penthouse* magazines. Hugh Heffner did not originate sex and pleasure; God did. Yet, because of man's evil mind, God-given attributes have been corrupted. This has occurred, I believe, because the church has been silent on such issues and Satan has gained ground. Yet, through the books I write, I hope I can open the eyes of Christians and make them aware of the good in marriage coitus. It should not be feared, but rather, understood and embraced within the boundaries of holy matrimony.

Reference
1. Sproul, R.C. Intimate Marriage—Sexual Problems in Marriage: Ligonier Ministries – DVD Collection. 1995
2. Fulbright, Yvonne K. <u>SEX YOUR WAY TO BETTER HEALTH: A DOZEN REASONS WHY YOU SHOULD HAVE SEX TONIGHT</u>. 2007. FOXNEWS. December 17, 2007.<http://www.foxnews.com/story/0,2933,317189,00.html>

THE GOLDEN RULE

The Golden Rule

This one simple rule can and will save and preserve any marriage. The rule is simple: Do unto others, as you would have them do unto you. In putting this rule into practice consistently, your marriage will get better. Husbands have been guilty of using the rule only when they want sex. This is not the way to engage the Golden rule. In fact, we need to use this rule all the time. When you use the rule all the time, it becomes a habit. This is one good habit to have in place.

When you put others before yourself, you are always blessed. The question we must all ask ourselves is: Will I learn from Christ's example of how much He loved others? Christ gave His life to bless others. Men especially must go about this program in the same way. Men must fight the instinct to please only self. Husbands must turn around and please their spouse to the best of his ability. Do unto others, as you would have them do unto you.

Men, take the time to use the rule not only when you are horny. Face reality and say," I must be nice to my wife because I want her to be nice to me always and everyday of our lives." Women have ways of knowing your intentions. If the Golden Rule is only in place when you want to have a golden time (sex), you are not doing well by the Golden Rule. The Golden Rule does not look for rewards. The Golden Rule works without rewards. The Golden Rule is the closest thing to Agape love on earth because you do the right thing without looking for a particular reward. Do unto others, as you would have them do unto you.

The Golden Rule, however, can tarnish if you are not careful. A tarnished rule is when you do right because you are forced into it, and the tarnish happens when one dominates the other or becomes a control freak. When the Golden Rule is not followed, other deviations come into play. When you see the tarnished rule in play, marriage becomes a curse instead of a blessing. Without the Golden Rule, you have tarnished attitudes.

I believe that if the Golden Rule is not followed correctly, it is discolored and stained. At its basest, everything that couples say to each other just blows up in flames. There is no structure following a tarnished rule. As soon as you build something, the marriage comes back down because the marriage is made of flawed (tarnished) material. Do unto others as you would have them do unto you.

The Golden Rule becomes stained and sullied quickly when couples do not try to keep the fire burning. Yes, this includes Christian couples as well (See the website *marriageromance.com* for pointers on ways couples can increase love and romance and keep it on the front burner instead of the back burner.) If you do not keep the romance going, the house will burn down.

We have seen in our forests how quickly huge and raging fires start, and the same is true with a marriage based on dried and rotted wood. In essence, if you do not work on the

Golden Rule, failure will rule all the aspects of your life.

I think a big issue for Christians is that some keep the Golden Rule in church but not at home. You cannot have different rules for the different aspects of your life. In terms of the Golden Rule, it is either one way or no way. A Christian spouse cannot apply the Golden Rule to fellow Christians and fail to apply it to his or her spouse. This is a form of hypocrisy.

It not just <u>doing</u> the Golden Rule but also <u>keeping</u> the Golden Rule. This is the challenge that each of us must face. Can we continue this philosophy throughout our lives as a married couple? Even when I want to have sex, I must remember the Golden Rule. I must not touch my spouse my way, but I must touch her in her way. Do unto others, as you would have them do unto you.

Let me explain. Say for example, that one person in the marriage has an unusual urge or one person in the marriage may want sex more and in different variations than the other. Whoever has the unusual urge must not badger or pressure the spouse to conform. Rather, the individual must pursue the spouse following the Golden Rule. What gets couples into trouble is when the spouse with the urge performs a dance to get his spouse in the mood. He errs by going there on his own. The other spouse is neither involved nor impressed; the spouse with the urge is hurt and bewildered. Then no one gets sex, and now you have two frustrated people in bed. The Golden Rule is in action when, if one spouse needs a certain something before sex, that spouse's needs are met.

You cannot reach your goals with a wooden attitude. You must reach your spouse with a Golden attitude. Once in bed, the Golden Rule still applies. You give your wife the type of loving she needs according to her needs. Yes, men, you compromise in the marriage and this shows when couples share the Golden Rule.

You cannot expect a spouse to enjoy sex when the Golden Rule is not enforced. Speaking of 'enforced,' if couples have to beg and beat each other up to apply the Golden Rule, then something is surely wrong and the Golden Rule has lost its market value in this home. The Golden Rule applies in sex when married couples willingly submit in love to one another. Do unto others, as you would have them do unto you.

There is no substitute for this. The Golden Rule is in place when couples engage in loving submission to one another. Anything different asks for trouble down the road. You cannot continue in any other vein and expect to have great sex and a great marriage. The Golden Rule works unbelievably in and outside of the bedroom. You must believe this for it to work. Faith without deeds is a dead end. You must come to grips with this rule and apply it generously to the marriage. You cannot apply the Golden Rule lightly. You must give considerable amounts of love and apply the rule liberally. Yes, there will be times when the wife or husband will give her/his best and the spouse does not return that level of emotion.

Remember, the Golden Rule is not based on what the other person does. It is solely based on what the initiator does. You must conduct yourself without looking for results. We apply the Golden Rule to our spouse not to get sex, not to get medals, but because my savior has given me the example to follow. As Jesus told His disciples to follow Him, we must follow Christ in this great aspect of life called love. The only way to survive is having the Golden Rule rooted in your relationship with your spouse. Do unto others, as you would have them do unto you.

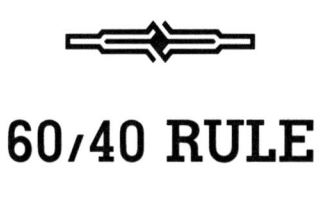

60/40 RULE

60/40 Rule

Many couples have no idea how much their parents have affected them both negatively and positively.

Before you walk down the aisle and say, "I do," your parents have already taught you a way of thinking about and acting in marriage. Be aware of this and be careful. In other words, before you build a marriage you must see, interpret, and adjust the things you saw as a child—how your parents interacted within the marriage. Regardless if you grew up in a traditional or nontraditional household, you will still have internal issues to debate. Ideally, you will wrestle with these issues BEFORE you walk down the aisle. Too many times, married couples fight unresolved battles inherited from their parents.

You would be surprised at how automatically you become your father or mother during an argument. Many couples do this because they: 1) do what they learned as children and 2) are more comfortable or at ease acting like their role models—father or mother—in difficult times. We fail to understand that just as PHYSICAL attributes (nose, eyes, and hairline) link families together, so do

EMOTIONAL attributes link families together.

The EMOTIONAL attributes are as critical as the PHYSICAL attributes. Just as you cannot deny physical similarities in your family, you cannot deny emotional similarities. In fact, the more you deny, the more you will blame your spouse. There is no denying this point. Instead of speaking to your spouse, you will be speaking to Mom or Dad.

Let me explain. As children, we could not respond to our parents when they fought. While the sparks flew, you were probably in your room wishing you could defend either mom or dad but you could not. So, fast-forward to your marriage. You have the fights, arguments, and pain of your parents in your brain. When your spouse says a word that links you to your childhood, without knowing it, you will speak to the past and not the present. This is the 60/40 Rule at work.

Couples can work on their own issues (40%) but until they resolve the past parental issues (60%), the married couple will think they are working on themselves in the present when, in reality, they are trying to resolve the parents' pain. This is very important for couples to be aware of, figure out, and eventually resolve.

Corporate America uses the 80/20 rule. It says 20% of customers create 80% of the revenue that comes into the business. Well, a similar concept works in relationships, but in a different way. You inherit 60% of all fights and disagreements from your parents, and you get 40% of your issues from your own individual proclivities. However, since 60% is greater than 40%, it makes sense to tackle the bigger percentage first. Face the giant (60%) and the dwarf (40%) will not cause a major issue for you. **Maybe this explains why parents understand when**

their kids divorce—they see similarities in their marriage and that of their own kids. Again, this is very important for couples to become aware of, figure out, and resolve.

We have all heard of haunted houses. (I still wrestle with the idea.) I do, however, believe in emotional, haunted marriages. The houses are marriages haunted by emotions or issues of the past. Together you have haunted couples. In addition, let me say quickly, as a Christian, I do believe in exorcising demons. But marriages are filled with haunted issues from the past, not demons. At times, demons can be misinterpreted as past emotional issues and vice versa.

The key is, before you think *demon,* think *parents.* Before you engage your spouse in a heated discussion, look to the sins of Mom and Dad. Think about what you do not like about your spouse. First, see if you detect any similarities that stem from your experience with your parents. In fact, before you condemn your spouse, first condemn your parents for any bad traits they passed down to you. Before criticizing your spouse, see if you should instead criticize your parents.

As humans who deal daily with emotional issues, we must constantly fight. The emotional affects us more than the physical because we can quickly put our hands on the physical. The emotional issues are more elusive, and, most of the time, emotional issues appear when we least expect them.

In fact, they resemble little time bombs waiting to go off. Bombs are created and buried early in our lives, from the ages 2 to 10; then, when we become teenagers, the bomb starts to tick. Unless the bomb is dismantled, it may just blow up later, during marriage.

Many people will confess that the most aggravation

they ever felt occurred not in single life, but in married life. Why? Because married life often resembles the war zone, we saw as kids. Therefore, it makes sense that arguments with your spouse will remind you of the war zone you lived in as a kid. When you experienced it as a child, you interpreted this in your childlike mind. Your mind imprinted the fights, dissected them, and programmed them.

Yet now, as an adult, you should dissect the program. Often, when we grow up, we still carry our childlike interpretation. So when issues arise with our own spouse we have a childish, not adult, reaction and interpretation.

How do you flip this switch? Simply, you deal with issues before marriage instead of after marriage. You must be honest about your parents and not deny their DNA within you. When we really look in the mirror directly and honestly, we see 60% of our parents. Many spouses turn a devil-parent into a deity.

We must be aware of this and be careful to avoid it. I have seen many grown kids speak only about the good of their parents and never the negative. This issue continues the pain of a grown child who will not reconcile the bad things that they saw.

When that spouse does not reconcile these memories and emotions, he or she will place ALL the blame on the spouse. Once you recognize the 60% you carry with you into the marriage from your family experiences, you must destroy the curse. I remember the *Son of Dracula* movies, where the lead actor inherited the curse of the father. He knew his tendencies and so must we. We must know when we have these triggers, and we must take a proactive approach toward these mysteries in our lives.

Sometimes at the end of a horror movie, the son kills himself to save others from his curse and to put an end to it. This idea of killing ourselves or part of ourselves is unacceptable and will not work; your DNA is your DNA. You cannot change this, but you can control the negative DNA. In another movie, *The Hulk*, the protagonist tried to control his emotions, and, in the end, he did. So must we. You cannot destroy who you are.

Therefore, the next best thing is to have awareness and control and maintain (with the help of God of course). The danger is living your whole life trying to kill something that will NEVER die. Therefore, we must change the repeating motif. We must change the tenor of how we deal with these issues from our parents. We must be aware, monitor this, and change the curse.

For those spouses who do not know their parents, you must inquire and find answers to your questions. It will be a relief to know WHY you do WHAT you do. Many couples are in the dark in this territory. Again, when you see how you get from happiness to pain, then you know your foundation. So, if you were adopted or never knew your father or mother such attitudes must change. You must know them to control them.

After discovering your parents' demons, you can deal with your own. Again, it is 60% your parents and 40% your marriage. When you learn to tackle your parents' demons, you can tackle your own. In my opinion, the parents' demon always weighs heavier than the child's own demon. Once you deal with it, then you inherit the power to deal with your demon. The key is to own what is yours; what belongs to your parents, THEY get to keep. Confusing the two will cause problems and headaches down the road.

Consider this even more profound thought: if YOU do not break the cycle, you will hand it down to your kids. This is the tragedy of the drama. As you watched your parents, your children watch and track you. As you learned from Mom and Dad, so will your children. By controlling the demon through prayer and honesty, by being a role model, you train your child in how to combat the demons. If you do not combat the demon, it will only increase for the next generation. The goal is not to let the next generation take on your sins. If anything, as parents our job is to control the demons that your children will face one day in their own marriages. At best, you want to pass on a positive 60%.

FORGIVENESS

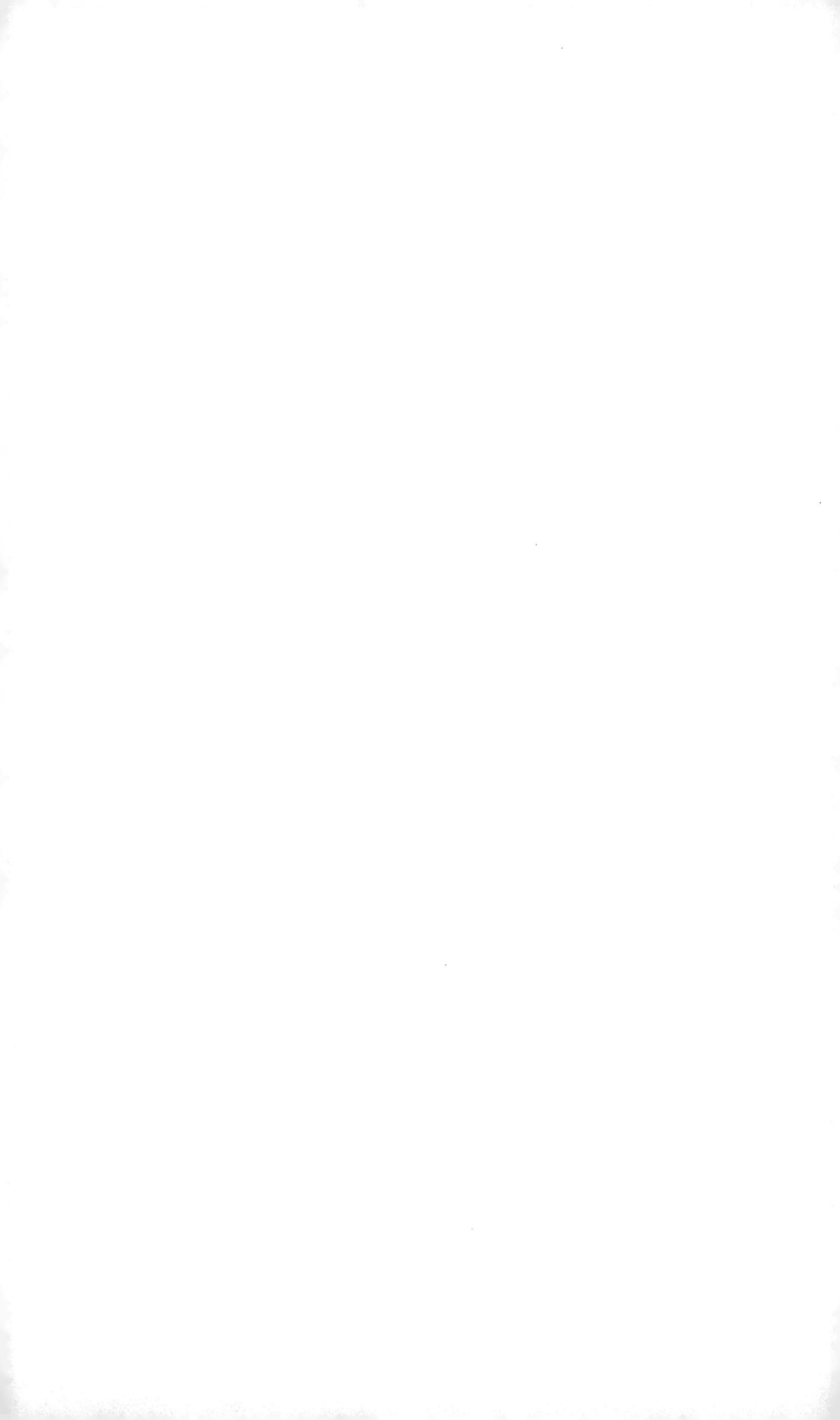

FORGIVENESS

For married couples to have great sensual experiences, they MUST know great forgiveness. This is especially true among Christian married couples. For reasons that only God can explain, some Christian couples are so self-righteous toward each other, they trip over their self-righteous robes. As individuals, they do not see their own sins, but they can see the sins of their mates extremely well. They can point out the offenses of their mate and never even see their own wrongs in the relationship.

Unless couples are willing to forgive, there will be no bedroom action at all. When you do not forgive, you only stay in the mess; a mess that goes unclean will start to stink up the area. Many couples cannot enjoy great sex because they will not forgive each other. Yes, it may take some counseling, but hear me out. If you expect to stay in a marriage, why beat up yourself and your spouse in the process? If you expect to stay with each other, you might as well get beyond yourself, forgive one another, and let the love flow.

On a very powerful note, most unwillingness to forgive

stems from an individual not forgiving himself or herself for past mistakes. For a couple to survive, they must first survive themselves. In other words, they must reconcile their own pasts before they can reconcile with each other. This is a powerful point that only some couples get. Once you deal with YOU, then you can deal with your mate.

Many couples trip over themselves because they stay in the frigid climate of non-forgiveness; when you stay in the climate of non-forgiveness, you will become like the climate of non-forgiveness—cold and miserable. As Christians especially, this should be an easy lesson to learn because God, through Christ, forgave us. So it goes, if God forgave us, we should follow that example and forgive our mates.

Let's be honest: no one, and I mean no one, can lay claim to perfection. No one is born without sin. In a relationship, contentious issues arise. But if a Christian couple realizes how God forgave them, they then must turn that around and forgive their mates. Space limitations do not permit me to dive into forgiveness in depth. However, as a good Bible study, I suggest couples find every reference on forgiveness in the Bible and read it over. You will find some powerful points.

However, when it comes to cheating, well, this may take some counseling—along with forgiveness. Remember, take your time and get back to one another; it will work out in the end. The bottom line is this: if you do not forgive, you cannot love each other. You cannot take those moments and move each other to a higher point of loving. IF you want more sex, then you have to forgive more.

HOME FIRST; MINISTRY SECOND

Home First; Ministry Second

Due to just plain ignorance, many spiritual leaders have made their ministry a priority and have let their marriages spoil. When I first married, I heard from and believed many when they told me if I took care of God's business, He would take care of mine (marriage). However, last I checked the Holy Ghost only once came down from Heaven and impregnated the Virgin Mary. I do not want to go too deeply into this, but no man wants another man taking care of his business, especially in the bedroom. I must take care of my priority, which is my family.

Because many preachers have not adopted this stance of family first, many preachers' kids want nothing to do with the church. They saw that Mom, Dad, or both failed to give attention to the family. Therefore, by the time the kid becomes of age, he or she had nothing to do with the church. Men and women of God, we must take care of our priorities. The first priority that God gave man was not the ministry. The first priority was the family.

Nowhere do I see Adam moving from home to the pulpit. He kept his priorities straight. Adam's priority, before Eve, was God; yet, after Eve, things changed. To continue on this point about ministry priority, far too many times the church becomes the "other woman" or the "other man" in a relationship. The married minister is not supposed to give all his or her time to the church. That person is not supposed to love the church more than the home. The man or woman of God should not give more to the church in love, emotion, and finances without loving his family first.

I have heard of pastors giving up everything to keep the church alive while the family suffered. I have even heard a preacher say proudly that he only had 1 cent in his pocket. Later that preacher's family had to hunt to get the money together to bury him. I even heard one bishop say that he was not going to leave his family any money because he could not spend it. He did not think about his family first; he thought about the church more. This is wrong and a downright sin. You cannot love the church and hate your family.

Too many times the husband or wife put all their energy into the church to avoid going home. This is simply bad theology. In fact, Paul said that a bishop should have his home in order before assuming the role of a bishop (I Timothy chapter 3 and verse 4). I think Paul asked: how can you preach the gospel and not have your own home in order? You cannot.

What sense does it make to teach the masses and not teach your own children? You have to have the right order. Anything out of order will cause confusion. This is what I often see happening within the body of Christ: a whole lot of confusion with ministers trying to get to God but stepping over their own kids in the process of doing so. It is very tempting to leave home for church. It is tempting when your wife reacts angrily after you have told her God has lead you to a revival or an event in another city, state, or country. Once I heard an evangelist brag that he had not been home in six months as he traveled to preach the Lord's Word.

My brother or sister, with that spirit you help nobody. You are only running away from your responsibilities. We see that soldiers have a hard time readjusting to home life because they have been away so long. It is the same issue with pastors, evangelists, and anyone who stays away from home while following a calling.

We must keep things in order to avoid a train wreck. When you do not love your spouse, you will have hell to pay down the road. I have seen too many men wear the bishop's ring and not his or her own wedding ring. How can you say you love your wife and not wear your wedding ring? That makes no sense to me, at all. You go, preach, and wear other rings on your fingers, but not your wedding ring. Something is wrong with that. Dress it up as you want, but, dear sir, you are not married to the church. Those in ministry are not married to God. The church is married to Christ, but the man is married to the wife and vice versa.

You cannot continue such a trend and expect a blessed life. How can we minister to the men and women in our churches when we do not set examples? There are too many graves of pastors who have died young because they gave more to the church than to the home. Brothers and sisters, there are things that a spouse will do for you that a church will never and should not do for you. How can a wife give love to her husband when there is no love coming her way? There is no way a husband can bless a wife if she never blesses her husband. The order of wife/husband and church must be kept and honored.

We cannot forget that Adam's first job was at home and not at church. We get it mixed up sometimes in our churches. It is easy to be successful in business, and for the most part at your church, but to be successful in your home is another beast. For too long, the rule of success has been the size of your church or how much money you have in the bank, but we must turn the corner, say that success is measured by family, and love in the household. My success is defined by the good loving that I give to my spouse in and outside the bedroom.

Some preachers have made the church their mistress or paramour. This is wrong on several fronts. Many go on long revival tours just to love the church more than their spouses. Loving God takes top priority over everything, but loving your church does not come in second. Loving your spouse and family comes first after God. Yet many preachers make love to the church, spend all their time in church, and never give the wife or family their love and share. By the time they get home from doing the "Lord's Work" they are dog-tired and have no energy to fulfill their promise to spouse and family.

This is keeping a mistress, and such behavior cannot be tolerated. Some preachers have committed adultery from a spiritual point of view by giving the church more time than the spouse. The church can be very addicting because of the praise and honor received from the congregation and others. Like nymphets who sang to the sailors to get them to destroy their boats, the faithful praise to some preachers makes them forget about their duty to their families. This, sir and madam, is wrong.

Your first priority is to your family and providing for

them. Your family does not deserve leftovers. When you do not give them quality time and effort, then you are not really giving your family prime time. Anything less than prime time, as it relates to your wife or husband, is like having an affair.

The Word of God says that to be a bishop you must be the husband of one wife. Paul says if you want to be a bishop, you must be married to one wife. So, if marriage is part of the requirement, then why not proudly wear your wedding ring and honor the biggest qualification to be a bishop? I hear you saying, "She does not love me," and I say to you she probably cannot stand you because you give her neither time nor patience.

You do not give her quality time and no quality time means NO sensual pleasure in the marriage bed. We must be able to marry the spiritual and sensual at the same time. Yes, pastor, the church loves you but your wife does not. You cannot just please your church. Your spouse must be taken care of first. She must know that you have your pecking order correct: home and then church.

This issue must be addressed. Too many popular pastors divorce their wives and get new ones within a year. How can ministers tell their congregation to hold on when they themselves do not hold on? I know these days are hard for pastors, but we cannot abandon the original ship called marriage. I must take this further in reference to preachers and their homes before I conclude this chapter.

Many preachers know how to preach to their wives but do not have a clue about making love to them. We have a host of pastors who know how to give book, chapter, and verse on a biblical topic, but know little about giving their wives sexual pleasure. Lord help us!

If the husband were more understanding and loving, he

would not need to recite book, chapter, and verse because his life would be a living testimony. The love, patience, and orgasms that a preacher gives to his wife speak volumes of a husband. I know, Preacher, your spouse can get on your nerves. Sometimes he/she talks about church more than sex and you, but you must endure because you are married to your spouse and not the church.

A real man will keep his member home and work it out with his wife both in and outside the bedroom. Preachers preach love, mercy, forgiveness, and sex to your wife, and you will be surprised at the "growth" of your ministry in and out of the bedroom.

Reference
Focus on the Family. The Parsonage.
<http://www.parsonage.org/>

IF HE STOPS, WHAT WILL YOU DO, WIVES?

If He Stops, What Will You Do, Wives?

It is unfair and wrong for a wife to tell her man to stop a sexual vice and then withhold sex from him when he decides to make the wife his only sexual desire. I understand, wives, it may take a while for you to forgive him and trust him, but after a while, if you see his dedication, then you must turn the page. Some wives just have no heart. For a wife to turn down requests for sex and not make herself sexually available to her husband is just plain wrong once the change in the husband is permanent. Do I dare ask, did he turn to a sexual vice because you turned off the sexual power that God gave you? I do not justify any wrong of the husband toward a wife, but if the husband makes the change, the wife must relent.

I have counseled many wives who wanted their husbands to stop sexual vices, but after the man stopped his vice, some of the wives did nothing, and I mean nothing. In fact, some of them became less sexual, and, on top of that, dared the husband to perform the sexual vice again. This does not compute. This will not work.

Many wives first do not realize the pull their husbands have concerning sex. In Shaunti Feldhahnon's book, *For Women Only: What You Need to Know about the Inner Lives of Men* (2004) she writes:

On each survey and in my random interviews around the country, an urgent theme emerged: Men want more sex than they are getting. And what's more, they believe that the women who love them don't seem to realize that this is a crisis – not only for the man, but for the relationship.[1]

Some husbands when they are not satisfied turn to sexual vices. Sexual vices are things that disgust the wife that a husband may do by himself without the wife. I am saying, wives, if you want your man to stop sexual vices that do not include you, then you have to step up your game—especially after, he cleans up his act. Yes, that means you have to become more aggressive toward your husband sexually.

He wants you to come after him more and not beg you for sex every night. You cannot continue to beat him up when he desires you after he says, "I will stop the sexual vices." Some wives ask, "If I become more sexual what is he going to do?"

Wives, I prophecy you WILL have a new man in your life because instead of going off on his sexual vices, he will come after you.24/7. Yes, I said 24/7. As men do not comprehend a woman's desire and need to communicate, nor does a wife understand her husband's capacity to have sex. Just as a wife wants the husband available 24/7 for open communication, the husband wants the wife available 24/7 for sex with him. The wife wants the communication her way. A husband wants the sex his way, as well. Wives, you want variety in your communication, so do husbands want variety in sex.

For religious people who say "Jesus!" to the above, I say, "Wrong!" You do not say "Jesus!" when you hunger or want to go to the bathroom, do you? As eating is human, so is sex in a marriage. Simply desires need to be meet. Wives, you do not call it nasty when you eat a full meal, so why call your husband crazy or nasty when he desires to eat from your 'plate'.

When he needs you to touch, massage, or play with his member, do not get crazy and refuse him; he is just putting all his energy into you. Wives, can you handle the truth of your husband's sexual libidos? It is alive and well, and if you want your man to stop all sexual vices, you have to step up. This means getting sexier for him at home. It means talking sexually to your husband.

It means giving him his daily diet of sexual passion as he gives you a daily diet of companionship and communication. As surely as a wife needs her daily diet of communication, so does a husband need a daily diet of sex in his life.

If you get your husband to stop his sexual vices, he may turn to you for sex EIGHT or more times during the week.

In addition, no, you cannot say, "If you want it, it's here." That is just not enough. Just as you go to the store to buy clothing, your husband wants you to come to his store (penis) and take care of him. Can you handle his coming to you for quickies or other forms of sex on a daily basis? Please do not get me wrong, a marriage does not live by quickies alone. There needs to be romance in the relationship, but you cannot deny quickies either.

Wife, your man is a sexual emotional creature, and you are not going to wish away his desire once he stops sexual vices.

Again Shaunti Feldhahnon's writes:

Although popular opinion portrays males as one giant sex gland with no emotions attached, that is the furtherest thing from the truth. But because men don't tend to describe their sexual needs in emotional terms, we women may not realize that.

Due to hidden emotions, men are afraid of the issues that may arise when they give up a sexual vice for their wife. I believe most men want to please their wives, but husbands often fear that when they drop their sexual vices, they do not know what they will get in return. I know he is supposed to stop because he is a Christian man. However, wives, he is still a man with strong desires.

Yes, God will bless him, but his desires must still be met; he still needs your love - your physical love. In addition, just as you want your husband to meet your desires, you must meet his.

I must quickly say though, no spouse can meet ALL the desires of the respective spouse. Only God can meet such desires. Only God can move an individual to full compassion. With that being said, let God meet all your desires, and let your spouse be the frosting on the cake.

Prayer is good; but prayer will not wish away a man's natural sexual desires. You must take the journey with him. You cannot send him on the journey by himself. You cannot tell your husband, "Ok, you stopped your sexual vices, so now you walk the journey all alone." That is not going to work. If you want your man to stop his sexual vices, walk with him in this journey.

In addition, the journey is more than just holding hands—it is rocking his world. It is making him feel like a king in the bedroom. It is having fun with your husband sexually and not acting like a board. It is letting yourself go in his arms as you direct him to think about you first and not his sexual vice. Yes, wives, husband desire a lot of sex, but when you communicate your desire for him, he will pull back from vices and go to you, especially if he is a good man.

Wives, be careful what you wish for. <u>If you want him to stop, you must begin</u>. I will say that again: if you want your husband to stop doing sexual things by himself, then you must step up your sexual game and come after him. Yes, I said it. You must become more sexually active. I understand there are kids around, but you know how to show your husband a small window of a thigh, a leg, and a breast every now and then. Wife you know what your husband likes. **Wives YOU MUST reward your man for being totally yours sexually.**

I must say, once you take that road with your husband, there is no turning back. You cannot keep telling him, "I have a headache." You cannot keep rejecting him in the bedroom. You must also be a happy and engaged partner in the sexual experience. Do not just stand there. You have to dig deep and get involved with your husband.

If anything will make a man angry, it's when a wife says "Come to me," or "Stop your sexual vices so I can be your sexual creature," but then she does just the opposite. That is a fight that is waiting to happen, and yes, emotions are going to be hurt and destroyed over this. <u>Wives, if you tell him to STOP other sexual vices, you have to also tell him to GO by loving him sensually</u>.

In other words, tell him to come to you on a daily basis. I am not suggesting that he no longer has to communicate with you anymore or that you become his sexual slave, but you will elevate your sexual involvement with your husband.

Sometimes the wife has more sexual needs than the man. If this is your plight men, thank God, and step up your game to your wife's needs. The bottom line is: whoever has the habit that is not good for the marriage must RESOLVE, but the other spouse must wake up and fulfill the other needs to the brim.

What couples do in the bedroom is up to them. I will not tell a couple what not to do with the exception of adultery. However, if a wife wants to tell a husband not to go elsewhere, then that means she is going to do it for him; boy, that sounds good to any man.

In other words, wives, you will help compensate for what you told him to stop doing. This is really the meaning of Eve's role. She was an aide to Adam. Wife, if you want your husband to stop his sexual vices, decide if you will be an aide or an enemy when it comes to the bedroom. Again, if you decide to be an aide, your husband then should not have to remind you of sexually favors you promised him.

In addition, on the subject of strip clubs, wives do not understand that when it comes to sex, if their husband is not satisfied sexually, he can seem to be like an untamed animal that may go to the strip club. Since you do not want him there, do things to suggest to him to stay home. Let me say that before going further I do not suggest strip clubs to any couple.

In order to deal with this issue if he is a faithful man, is to create your own strip show at home. By doing this, you take his passion and bring it home.

Some wives are very quick to tell their husbands how lazy they are in the kitchen/house chores, and lack good communication but these same women may be lazy in the bedroom.

Both husband and wife must work together to bring about harmony so that going to other vices or venues of sex is not an option.

Remember, people go out and get what they do not perceive what they have at home. In other words, if you satisfy your spouse in the bedroom, he will not have the need to want to go to the strip.

Wives, as you want your husband to cater to your needs when it comes to communication and 'mall shopping' just do the same in the sex department and he will have no need to go out and watch a stripper because he has one at home.

Some how married couples must go after each other needs to take away negative choices of their mate. When you do this, the mate who is going out has no excuse because she or he is getting their needs met at home.

Wives, if your husband is calling you a woman that rides a broom turn that broom into a pole and see the changes in him after of course he makes constant and consistent changes within himself.

REFERENCE
1. Feldhahn, Shaunti. <u>For Women Only: What You Need to Know about the Inner Lives of Men</u>. Multnomah Books, 2004.

SEEDS OF DIVORCE

Seeds of Divorce

Because of the misguided goals of some preachers, divorce has taken a front pew in church. Marriage has lost its high standards, even in the pulpit. Preachers and pastors now divorce their wives at alarming rates, without regard to how it affects the body of Christ. To be honest, the reason for high divorce rates is the love of the flesh. Pastors come home expecting their wives to treat them like the women at their local churches, and when the wives do not give them "glory and praise," they justify finding another person.

No marriage is perfect. However, to go out and find another physical body to have sex with is outright wrong. If the church does not uphold the standard of marriage, how can we expect the world to follow suit? Throughout history, some very powerful men in great Pentecostal denominations have divorced or cheated on their wives.

I know many Pentecostal men and preachers who do not even wear a wedding ring. I personally have great issues with such customs. Preachers perform the marriage ceremony and tell the couple to exchange rings. Yet the same married preacher who officiates at the ceremony does not wear a ring himself. Something is wrong with this situation, and the seeds of doubt are planted.

Some men and women grow up as a PK (pastor's kid) and see their fathers being unfaithful to their mothers during the marriage. What can you expect down the road? If the father cannot keep his pants on for his wife exclusively, what seeds is he planting in the home? I am not calling on men to be perfect. I am calling on men to be honest and faithful to the person God has given them. It is easy to have many women; it is harder to be loved and love by only one. Yet, because of these divorce seeds, those who do stay in the marriage are surrounded by such negative actions and attributes that unless a married couple is strong they will have no sensual coitus.

I must stop and say that if the sex is not sensual, it is not sex. Unless some sweat and love happens and clean sheets are needed every now and then, the sex is not sex. Even for those older couples, the same thing applies. If you are just going through the motions to quiet your spouse, you are not having sex. It has evolved to legal prostitution within your own home—legal prostitution when Christian couples just has sex without passion or love. They are just doing the deed. We have to do better in the body of Christ.

I know your wife is big, and I know your husband looks pregnant (he has a big belly), but couples must find a way to get the passion back. Without passion, the marriage will turn bitter or the seeds of divorce will grow and before you know it, there will be great separation. No longer will you two have love. You will have issues on top of issues. Rather, when you have great sex, issues are relieved – at least for the minute or half hour. Again, if there is no love or passion, divorce will walk in.

Divorce is a weed. If you do not keep up the garden, the weeds will grow. Before you know it, you will have more weeds than flowers. Sex is like flowers. With the absence of sex, you will get weeds. Flowers need much attention. Sex between couples needs much attention. Communication between couples needs much attention; these things will not just happen on their own. You must attend to them.

If you do not attend to lovemaking, the weeds will come up. In addition, yes sir, your wife may not be into sex, but I GUARANTEE you, if you do not have sex, divorce will grow in the home. It may not be an actual, physical divorce; it may be an emotional divorce. If you do not fight for your marriage, such issues will come on you before you know it.

Furthermore, do not let bitter couples into your life. It just does not work. It will not work at all in any way. Find your own rhythm in the bedroom. Even if the music is off the beat, find your rhythm and stay with it. Michele Weiner Davis writes,

"People who are unhappy in their marriages often speak of feeling trapped. They yearn to be free from the tension, loneliness, constant arguments, or defending silence but worry that divorce may not be the right decision. After all, they took their martial vows seriously...They fear the unknown." (*The Divorce Remedy*, 2002)[1]

In fact, you have to find the rhythm again. Do not let chance be the factor; YOU must be the factor in finding the right steps to take to heal your relationship. Again, remember, with the seeds of divorce all around us, if couples do not take action, it will be taken against them. Without doubt, if couples do not fight to keep their ground, the weeds will continue to grow. This especially covers sex.

Reference
1. Davis, Michele Weiner. <u>The divorce remedy: The proven 7-step program for saving your marriage</u>. New York: Simon & Schuster, 2002

STIMULUS PACKAGE: SEX AS A TOOL—NOT AS A WEAPON

Stimulus Package: Sex as a Tool—Not as a Weapon

Too many men and women use sex as a weapon against their spouse. Such behavior can and will kill the relationship in the end. When a couple learns to use sex as a tool instead of a weapon, they go from being a simple couple to an educated and happy couple.

As I write this in 2009, America is in a recession and President Obama and Congress are trying to revive the economy through different measures. These measures include dealing with banks, sub prime loans, regulations, unemployment, and the list goes on. The point I am making is that the president is not sitting on his hands and HOPING things will get better. No sir, he is actively putting things in place to get the economy going again. If he does nothing, then America may never recover from a hole in which we find ourselves.

Well, marriages also need stimulus packages. For God, the stimulus package starts with love and forgiveness, but the kicker is sex. A couple needs to understand that at times in the marriage they need to do things differently to restart and re-energize things. In addition, let me say for the record, it does not matter who starts it, as long as it gets started.

Many times one person in a couple says, "I am tired of always doing things." Someone has to do something differently to keep the relationship going. The concept of stimulus means getting the party started—stimulating things. It means putting something into a system to get things moving along. This is what couples need to have in mind when they find themselves in the rut of doing nothing in their marriage.

Together they must find a way to get their marriage, and yes, their sex lives going again. If you do nothing it will surely die, but if you reach for the moon and get to the sun, at least you took a step in the right direction to save your marriage.

No marriage will survive without stimulus packages every now and then. Just do it for the sake of the relationship. This may include vacations, finding hobbies together, having sex in a hotel room, or countless other things couples can agree upon. Too many couples do nothing and expect something out of their marriage. This is the definition of crazy: when you do nothing and expect a great reward down the road.

President Obama said that he understands the results of the stimulus package will not be felt immediately, but at least, he is getting the party started. He is doing something now that will be felt later on. The husband and wife must not wait until the problem hits but must be proactive and go after the problem in their relationship instead of always being reactive to issues in their marriage.

For some couples, this may include counseling, and for others, it may include just getting away for a weekend. But, again, the smart couples will put something in place to get the ball rolling. They will not just look at the problem; rather, they will find solutions together to solve issues that may be affecting their marriage.

Infections that cause death in patients present a big problem for hospitals. The same can be said of couples that do not STIMULATE their marriage. They <u>must</u> interject something into their relationship before the infection of boredom and misery sets in. This does not include affairs or swinging. Couples must take the steps to keep things hot, heavy and fresh between the husband and wife, exclusively.

Before the government's stimulus package became law, it first had to be approved. This same concept applies to the marriage. Husband and wife must approve the stimulus package to get things started. They must first recognize the problem, and then they must find the solution together. For some couples the solution may be doing different things within the marriage that excite each other.

Christians, you will not be struck down on the spot if you do something together to spark sexual fireworks in your marriage. As long as it is agreed upon, have at it. If you are not comfortable with going places, then use the Internet. The only rule I offer is: never go to these places by yourself. I know you want to, husbands, but you had better not go without your wife. And, yes, the same goes for the wives. The temptation may be there, but remember, you are trying to find a stimulus package that will satisfy both of you.

Let us get back to the point of using sex as a tool and not a weapon. This is all a part of the stimulus package. There is power in having sex as a tool and not as a weapon. Many couples use sex as the first thing to do to punish their mate when offended. So, now, instead of sex giving pleasure, some mates use sex as a weapon to hurt and kill. Wait. I do not remember the marriage vows saying, "I will use sex as a weapon to hurt my mate." Neither do the vows say, "I will use sex to dispose of my spouse."

This is why sex should be used as tool. It should be used as a way to correct behavior. For example, while having sex, a wife could go over some things she desires from her husband. Yes, ladies, you have his full attention when you have sex. Therefore, she can say "I am having sex with you, why don't you do 'x, y, and z,' and I will do 'xxx, yyy, and zzz.' " You see the difference. You are now using sex as a reward system to reinforce behavior you like.

Take another example: Your husband is kissing you. You tell him, "If you want to go further later on in the day, I need this and that done first." Upon hearing this, a husband thinks, "If I do it, I get it." Again, this is using sex as a tool and not a weapon.

The word weapon gives the sensation of destruction and killing and hurting one another. But the word tool gives the sensation of FIXING something. This is why, when you use sex as a tool, you are using it to STIMULATE your marriage and not destroy it. After getting married, too many couples change the way they look at each other. This is not the answer. The answer is to love and appreciate one another to the point that there is a change that both husband and wife see. Again, the stimulus package will work if couples can look beyond themselves and see the goals of having a first-class, high-quality marriage.

Sometimes when couples argue, one will get mad and storm out of the room or yell at the other. How powerful would it be for a couple to love one another in the heat of a fight, instead of yelling at each other at the top of their lungs? This ugly arguing and carrying on fails to solve the issue, and at what price? How about when an issue comes up, you try saying, "Baby, instead of fighting, let's make love and think of ways to solve this issue while making love." You will be surprised that after orgasms, emotions like submission, mercy, and humility come to a couple.

I have already mentioned the power of sex when hormones are released. This just begs couples to use sex to help stimulate a marriage. Once again, I am not canceling or faulting communication; it is needed in a marriage. However, when you only communicate verbally and never physically stimulate each other, the fruit will die on the vine. The president is actively doing something to get things moving in the country. The same concept works for couples in the bedroom.

Husband, stimulate your wife. Wife, stimulate your husband. Do not just sit **there** and let your marriage die. Stimulate it back to health. This may include quickies or long-term romance. It may mean sitting down with each other going to a picnic. It may include doing things and going places. The key is doing something different to get something different out of the marriage.

You are stimulating, and, yes, when a husband sexually stimulates his wife, he WILL always get good results. Couples who find ways to keep their marriage hot and fresh have their own personal stimulus package.

We expect this country to recover, just as we expect the marriage to recover. We must put things in place to make it happen. Again, do something different. This could also include leaving something in the car or coming to the office unannounced in a nice outfit that says, "Wait till you get home tonight." Again, find something to stimulate your sex life and your marriage.

HAVE AN AFFAIR WITH YOUR SPOUSE
(LESSONS LEARNED FROM AFFAIRS & PROSTITUTES)

Have an Affair with Your Spouse

(Lessons Learned from Affairs & Prostitutes)

That is right, I said it. Married couples need to have affairs with EACH OTHER. For way too long, uncommitted, cheating, lying, unfaithful, and STD-carrying married couples have been having sex with persons who do not belong in their bedroom. Headlines after headlines contain stories of this person cheating with this person and that person cheating with that person. The time has come for committed married couples to take the excitement of an affair and place in into their marriage.

What I am proposing in this chapter is that couples admit that it has all right to have an affair, but with each other. The passion, power, and love can all be obtained legally. The secrets can be great. There would be no need for lying because it would be replaced with role-playing. Couples will just take that strand of affair (great sex and communication) and put it between them. The key is that this is a secret that only the two will know and share for a lifetime.

By having an affair with your spouse, you never get bored or come home to the same thing all the time. This ensures wedded bliss because every month you come home to a different wife or husband.

To pull this off, the couple must be of one accord. There can be no surprises. When you have an affair, you cannot surprise the other person by coming over without being told first, so the same thing works here. In fact, by having a marital affair with each other, you create and nurture communication between one another.

When you have **Affairs Within** or AW, communication is increased. This is needed because the first area you must discuss in order to have a successful AW is tell each other what is lacking in the marriage. Once you find what is lacking, you simply begin *to do*.

Wives and husbands, let me tell you that when your AW is happening, you do not think, you just act. For that moment, you escape—not from each other but to each other. As affairs are known for escapism, you are doing the same but with your loving and committed spouse.

Michael Bader of Alter Net conducted a study of men who visit prostitutes. His article was posted on March 14, 2008 under the title *"Why Men Do Stupid Things: The Psychological Appeal of Prostitutes"*.[1] In this article he states,

The appeal of hookers lies in the temporary psychic relief they supply to men struggling with conflicts about guilt and responsibility. Having studied the dynamics of sexual arousal for almost 15 years, and having treated dozens of men who find prostitutes irresistible, I have found that for the overwhelming majority of them, the appeal lies in the fact that, after payment is made, the woman is experienced as completely devoted to the man—to his pleasure, his satisfaction, his care, his happiness. The man does not have to please a prostitute, does not have to make her happy, and does not have to worry about her emotional needs or demands. He can give or take without the burden of reciprocity. He can be entirely selfish. He can be especially aggressive or especially passive, and not only is the woman not upset, she acts aroused. He is not responsible for her in any way. She is entirely focused on him. He is the center of the world. Now, of course, these interactions are scripted. The prostitute is acting. But it does not matter. For men who like to go to prostitutes, the illusion of authenticity is enough.

Do you see the reasons? We can learn to take these reasons and make them a learning tool to ensure outside affairs do not occur. Have you heard of learning from the enemy to defeat your enemy? I am trying to use the same concept in this chapter. Let us review and learn.

The woman is completely devoted to the man. She is entirely focused on him. He is the center of the world. This goes for wives and husbands as well. Indeed, during the affairs within and in ALL situations, you should feel that the other person is there for you. Complete devotion means needing and wanting one another. Yes, the needs may be selfish, but you are really saying to your partner on a given day that his or her wish is your command. During one Affair Within, the wife may get all her wishes, while on another night the husband gets all of his.

The man does not have to worry about her emotional needs or demands. He is not responsible for her in any way. Without a doubt, this cannot take place in a loving relationship at all times. A relationship is just the opposite of this. You are always listening and trying to deal with the demands of your mate. The job of both mates will simply be to minister love to each other. And let me add, if things are spoken during the Affairs Within, they stay within the Affairs Within.

If you start to question the fancies or requests outside the Affairs Within, this make an Affair Within feel like a regular day. On Affairs Within days, you will serve one another without looking for a need or demand to be met. Again, you must allow your spouse to be another person. However, you must not hold anything against them later on because you are giving each other a gift that should only be shared within the Affair Within.

He can give or take without the burden of reciprocity. He can be entirely selfish. On this special day, couples will fulfill each other's fantasies and be selfish. Again, it is just during the Affair Within that pleasure will be shared equally, but perhaps not simultaneously, between the wife and the husband. As a rule of thumb, you should remember that ladies come first. Furthermore, it is important to watch your attitudes toward each other. If you make it seem like pulling teeth, the Affair Within will not work. Freely given, freely received is the order of the day.

He can be especially aggressive or especially passive, and not only is the woman not upset, she acts aroused. Too many couples act like blow up dolls when they are having sex. This will stop during Affairs Within, and hopefully when the sex becomes great and powerful, it will carry over into non-AW days. The key is to be aroused when sexual activities happen. Let yourselves go and get involved in the stimulation (physical, emotional, or sexual). Throw caution to the wind.

During the Affairs Within, you are in an illusion, but it is one that is created together. An amusement park or a movie is an illusion. What I am prescribing to couples is that they make their own Never Land, a communicative, sensual place where they can escape from the world into each other's arms. In this land your mate is not asking for sex; rather, you are giving it without abandon. Again, this is not every day, but a place where you go occasionally together. You pray that such days will have residual value in the days to come.

During the Affairs Within, it is as if you embrace each other's dreams and concerns at the expense of your own desire. In other words, during these times, you deny yourself for a while and give your spouse his or her ultimate desire.

Do you know how many affairs happen and one party in the affair does not like say a certain sex act but they will do it to keep the person in their life. However, married couples, relating to the same sex act, have put a forbidden city on themselves as it relates to the same type (sex act) of bending and turning that the unfaithful give. This ought not to be.

If people in external affairs can twist and turn and accommodate one party just to keep them, how much more should married couples twist and turn and accommodate their legal mate on these Affair Within days? And who is to say that what happens during Affairs Within will not ultimately continue on non-AW days as well?

Michael Bader has some more interesting things to say about why men love prostitutes. He says, such men feel psychically weighed down by the belief that they are supposed to take care of women, that they have an obligation to make women happy, to please them. Such beliefs are often exaggerated and based on a belief and perception that women are high-maintenance, helpless, or disposed to be unhappy and dissatisfied... In real relationships, they feel that there is always a hidden quid pro quo that they can't get much unless they give a lot that they have to pay a high price for getting what they need. Of course, intimate relationships then suffer.

In this pressure cooker society, it is no wonder that couples are dying. There is no pressure during Affairs Within. Stress will be nonexistent during these times. The stress of trying will be gone and replaced by simply doing. During Affairs Within, husbands and wives will discover with fascination the wonder of the male and female gender. The notion of *quid pro quo* will go away and things will be done for the sake of the spouse.

Imagine an island where no bickering or complaining occurs. For some, this is a nonexistent island, but people in affairs are always positive and feeding such even though, their spoon is dirty. However, in a committed marriage, the spoon is clean but the food is tainted. Married couples must change this course somehow. I believe this can be done with occasional Affairs Within wherein the male and female genders are given equal footing.

Men are expected to understand women during pregnancies, menstrual cramps, and the way their wives communicate. I agree with this. Men are below the mark in understanding these things truly. Men will never experience having children, but we are expected to understand. It is important to note that the same goes for the wife with regard to understanding her husband and his sexual needs.

A wife will never understand the libido within her husband. However, I feel that society has been unfair to men. Men are expected to understand the needs of women, but women are not expected to step up their game in the sex department. During Affairs Within, both the husband

and wife will have equal footing. During these times, understanding will follow and appreciation for the female and male genders will be acknowledged.

Michael Bader continues, for these men, a prostitute is sought as a relationship in which the man can **"let go" and freely express** his most **selfish desires** without **feeling guilty and worried** about the effect of these desires on his partner.

The important aspect is that couples feel guilty when performing certain sex acts, yet in an illicit affair, either party does not feel guilt. Men and women cavort with each other and cheat on their wives and husbands without feeling any guilt. This must be stopped. It is wrong and ungodly for a husband or wife to feel dirty or guilty if they share their heart. The Bible says directly that the marriage bed is undefiled. If the bed is undefiled, then love and understanding should replace guilt.

During Affairs Within, couples say things to one another without feeling guilty about an act or a word that they really want to share. We must take back what God has given to married couples. God told us to be fruitful and multiply, but couples are guilt-ridden about saying and doing things they really want to do. It does not make sense to find an outside person with whom they may share these things.

We need to be able to share these feelings with our mate and feel free. It is wrong to share things with others that you cannot even express to your wife or husband. We must find other avenues whereby we may share these things without feeling guilty. Indeed, I think the way to do this is through Affairs Within.

For the record, I am not an advocate of adultery or the use of prostitutes. However, there are certain things we can learn from them to ensure that emotional and sensual hurdles are not holding married couples back. In Affairs Within, we learn from the wrong in order to increase and improve upon the right.

In all that I write, I am not encouraging men to threaten their wives with affairs or go to prostitutes. These actions do not have any place in a loving home. Trying to scare your wife into submission by saying, you are going somewhere else for sex and love is not an option. If anything, Affairs Within will pull you close to the one you love, and these exercises will encourage married couples to run into each other's arms instead of into the arms of strangers.

Veronica Monet, a former prostitute, wrote a book called *Sex Secrets of Escorts: Tips from a Pro* (2005)[2]. She was interviewed in the Seattle Post-Intelligencer paper and she shared insights about the sex trade and gave suggestions that can be applied within a more traditional home.

Kristin Dizon of the Seattle Post-Intelligencer explains Ms. Monet's distinctly different approach to making marriages work: by saying …And, yes, her book does include technical sex tips but says you also need good communication and negotiation skills. Written for "mainstream" married women, her book delves into a lot: **letting go of shame and body image issues**; self pampering and care that make you feel good and sexy; **learning to date your mate again**; setting healthy boundaries; **how to initiate sex and more**.

Ms. Monet asserts the very thing that professional marriage counselors have said throughout the ages: date each other and lose your shame with regard to your body. Every husband, especially during lovemaking, should let his wife know she is still beautiful. However, when you feel shame about your body, you feel shame about your sex life as well. Consequently, men should always applaud the beauty of their wives, even after they have had kids or they gain some weight. Our society has put much stock in the external and less in the internal. This is why married couples need to oppose such ideals and determine what works within their marriage in order to keep it together.

Notice the importance of initiating sex in the article. In the lives of prostitutes, this is the meat and potatoes of their occupation. Most of the time, people having outside affairs are having sex like rabbits. I propose couples do the same during their personal Affairs Within sessions. Affairs Within gives people the thrill of cheating while they are in fact cheating with each other. Husbands and wives take on roles that will hopefully spill over in their everyday lives. There is no guesswork when outside affairs go to a hotel room. It is going to be done, and that same mind frame should be part of your AW.

Kristin Dizon asked Ms. Monet the following question:

Q: A lot of women still wonder why men visit prostitutes. What is the answer?

A: First and foremost, men do not go to see therapists. They go to see prostitutes. So, when a man's feeling like something's lacking in his life, something's missing and he's not quite sure what it is… the prostitute or the mistress or the courtesan, or even the stripper, wind up being **confidantes**. The men are either too ashamed or too afraid or too protective of their ego or their power to make themselves that **vulnerable** to the people in their life. There is an exchange of cash, which gives the man the feeling that he is in control, so therefore, he can exercise no control…

Two words I highlighted above are "confidantes" and

"vulnerable." In other words, men get the feeling that their secrets are safe with a prostitute and they can rest without danger. Many, many couples do not have that kind of trust after the first couple of years of marriage. Husbands or wives cannot feel vulnerable because when they seek what they feel or want, they will be rejected.

During an Affairs Within, however, this is not the case. In fact, the man and woman will not only be open sexually but also be open from the point of view of communication; they will be able to share all and get things off their chests without feeling guilty. It is important to remember that this should also spill over into the marriage in the form of discussion. However, in Affairs Within, there is no discussion—just passion and acceptance of each other's plight and desires.

In my earlier book, *New Sheets*, I discuss how every man wants to be Samson in the lap of Delilah. Many men and women do not know how to take that first step into the island of vulnerability. When one is always hurt and put down, it becomes hard to become vulnerable, but it must be done. **Please understand that if you are not vulnerable to your spouse, you will become open or vulnerable to someone else.** Understand this point and open up, letting your spouse make you his or her confidante. Let them know that their secrets, desires, dreams, and concerns are safe with you.

Judges Chapter 4, Verses 18–21 tell of Jael, who killed Sisera, an enemy of Israel. He trusted a woman who in turn killed him. In an illicit affair, your secrets are in trouble and eventually something will 'die'. However, in the arms of your mate, this should not be the case. Spouses, please check yourselves even before an Affair Within. Can your mate tell you things without you coming down on them like a ton of bricks? If not, then you may drive your mate away to another. Once again, this stresses the importance of being open to your mate. If you cannot do this on a regular basis, at least do it during Affairs Within.

Kristin Dizon asked Ms. Monet another interesting question:

Q. So, what is your take on what makes men happy sexually?

A. I would say to women, stop worrying about making him happy. Make yourself happy. **Ironically, men are happiest when you are into your own selfish pleasure.** A lot of what men like about prostitutes is that prostitutes love their bodies and **they have sex with the lights on**. They flaunt themselves in a way that shows a lot of **sexual confidence**. They will **seduce the man**, and I do not mean by sitting across the room and batting their eyes. I mean actually pushing him down on the bed and having your way with him.

Before I comment on the above answer, I would like to point out that you will not be able to expect your wife to do anything during or after Affairs Within if you are not fully faithful and have NOT made an effort to be a better husband. A husband can NEVER, EVER ask his wife to be more sexually unless he has tried and completed the latter himself. If you are a good husband, then you can ask her to fulfill your desires and in turn fulfill her desires. Without such reciprocity, there will be no marriage.

Ms. Monet asserts that having the lights on, being sexually confident, and seductions are all wonderful to the ears of a husband with a high libido. When a woman lacks the confidence to seduce her husband, she gives off the vibe that she does not want her husband or that she hates sex. Let us be frank: if a wife does not like her body, she usually will not like sex. If she does not accept her body, she will not accept sex. The two go hand in hand. This is where a husband can act as a cheerleader for his wife and tell her how much he desires her. Upon doing so, she will hopefully rebuild her confidence in herself and her abilities to initiate and seduce her husband. However remember husbands, if you are an emotional terrorist, this is not going to happen.

Kristin Dizon continued asking Ms. Monet about this subject:

Q. What do you recommend for people with low libidos, or those who have just lost interest in sex?

A. The best advice... could be as simple as joining the gym. Exercise produces testosterone, and it also makes you feel better about your body, no matter what size and shape you are. **Just getting the blood flowing through everything gets you breathing and that can create a lot of sexual juice.** And, take better care of your body. . . You can start off with therapy, talk about how you feel about sex, journal about it, and start seeing what kind of feelings come up about it.

The major point being made here is that whatever is lacking is what needs to be fulfilled, and thus from the wicked we learn strategies to keep our marriage together.

Ms. Alexander, a relationship expert, writes the top ten reasons why men have affairs[3]

1. More sex (sometimes due to lack of sex in their relationship)
2. Sexual variety through different partners or different sexual experiences
3. To boost their ego or to feel special or attractive to the opposite sex

4. For the thrill of the chase
5. Opportunistic sex (if the opportunity occurs, they can't pass it up)
6. To sabotage their current relationship
7. Revenge (to get back at their partner for one reason or another)
8. A feeling of entitlement (the belief they are entitled because they work hard or are the bread winner)
9. Sexual addiction
10. To escape

It can be said that women seek a partner outside of marriage that will validate them and give them the emotional commitment that they do not get from their husbands. The top 7 reasons why women have affairs:[4]

1. To improve self-esteem (she enjoys the attention and compliments about her abilities and body)
2. New and varied sexual experience (she feels freer to experiment and explore with a lover than with her husband)
3. Emotional connection (she desires emotional closeness and intimacy)
4. Loneliness (she needs someone to talk with who will listen to her)
5. Deeper understanding of self (she learns from exploring her feelings and thoughts with someone who cares for her)
6. To feel younger and sexier (her lover's sexual desire for her makes her feel playful and free)
7. Fear of aging (she is afraid getting older will make her less attractive to men)

Husbands and wives should not fear theses lists but

learn from them. In other words, these are lists detailing what to do and what not to do to insure that these issues are being addressed in the relationship.

No doubt, the above lists should function as checklists of how couples are treating each other. This, of course, calls for honesty and openness to each other needs and wants WITHOUT getting offended. Once again, you are taking the power of affairs and placing it right in the center of your marriage.

When you learn from the list, you take away the urge to have an affair. For example, if a man's biggest issue is sex, then his wife will ensure that he is always satisfied. As for the wife, the husband will ensure that he is building and nurturing her self-esteem. If couples did this regularly, there would be no need—none whatsoever—for affairs. In fact, by having an AW, you continually and consistently meet each other's needs.

Couples who really love one another will learn from the negative to increase the positive. They will take the list and consistently see what is lacking in their lives before turning to a stranger.

They say most affairs happen within the first 7 years of a marriage or when someone within the marriage gets close to 50. Either way, instead of being reactive, be proactive about not having affairs. Have an affair, but have it with your spouse. Do not wait until the issue becomes a problem. Go for it now and tackle it to ensure peace and happiness in your home.

I cannot stress enough how fornicators and adulterers (whether homosexual or heterosexual) are enjoying something that in the very beginning was designed for faithful married heterosexual couples. The original design of marriage is to nurture and procreate. Since the creator is the designer, ONLY HE can change the design. God does not change because he is transcendent. What man has done is taken a gift that belongs to one group and applied it to all groups.

If someone buys property in a gated community, no one has a right to move in unless they are willing to pay the price to get in. This is the same issue with marriage and sex. Committed married couples belong in a gated community called sex, but others who have not paid the price want to enjoy this community. This is wrong.

Affairs happen because something is lacking in the relationship. The only way to deal with an affair is to find out what is lacking and meet the need. If you meet the need, then affairs will not take place. It is simple supply and demand. If you supply the demand of a spouse, there will be no affairs. If you control the supply of the demand, there will be no affairs in the house; this is simple marriage economics.

This system will work if the couple is willing to bend in order to ensure that affairs are only within. Of course, this system only works if the spouse is CURRENTLY FAITHFUL. I must say this again. You cannot come home and tell your wife you want an Affair Within when she just found out that you cheated for the first /second time. This will not work. However, for those who are in faithful relationships, you will see a number of benefits.

The constant theme is that whatever is lacking must be fulfilled, no questions asked. You are essentially telling your spouse that you are the one who is going to rock their world. You are the one who is going to support them, communicate with them, and make them feel important. No one else will have this responsibility but you. To simplify, spouses must supply each other's demands. This is the key to preventing affairs.

Infidelity is a serious thing and not to be taken lightly. The effects can last generations. All the words associated with affairs are painful, so I encourage couples to talk about their needs to each other without abandon. Adulteress, mistress, concubine, courtier, courtesan, doxy, cuckold (the husband of an unfaithful wife), and paramour are all words that carry the stigma of unfaithfulness.

Anyone who has been the victim of an affair will say that it is like having your heart ripped out because of the untruth that has occurred in the marriage. To stop the flow of pain from affairs, I encourage couples to have their own AW. This will include going to hotels for no reason at all and having great sex. Use role-playing to become another person and to let go of the inhibitions that challenge you in the real world.

Unbelievably, some prostitutes know their johns (husbands) better than their wives do, and this ought not to be. Affairs Within gives husbands and wives the opportunity to uncover secrets that they have been keeping from each other. When you have Affairs Within, there is no guilt or nasty comments. You are just enjoying your spouse by fulfilling their internal needs in a loving way. **It comes down to a very simple question: Would you not want your spouse to come to you rather than go to someone else?**

During Affairs Within, you can become the "bad boy" or "bad girl" for your mate's sake. You can let things go without abandoning each other. What happens is that when dating, we always want to put our best foot forward, and something's that same mind frame goes into a marriage when you don't want to show your spouse the worst or freak in you. During Affairs Within, you can let go of your inhibitions and enjoy the legal and godly passion you share with your spouse.

During an Affair Within, you reintroduce the art of teasing and flirting with one another. You may even want to bring back the garter from the wedding! What I am trying to do is create an adventure where the passion between husband and wife is reignited. There is no shame or guilt. You are touching, flirting, and doing those things that brought you together in the first place. If you had sex in the car when you were dating, then it is time to have sex in the garage now that you are married. WHATEVER you did to each other that kept your hands on the other person is EXACTLY what you need to do in an AW. Get the fire going and keep it burning no matter what.

Yes, time has a way of affecting the way we love our mates. Time has a way of coming after us and tearing down love and passion. It is up to each of us to put the pieces back together again. Of course, this is done with much communication and by strengthening the trust between the husband and wife. However, after such things are reestablished in the relationship, you can rock and roll with Affairs Within.

Do not be afraid to let yourself go in this setting. All over the country, American men and women are having affairs and there are no boundaries or holding back, so why in God's name should married couples hold back from something that God created for men and women who are married and committed to one another?

Enjoy your Affairs Within—ladies, get a wig. Men, get removable tattoos. Role-play to the fullest. Men should even take their socks off when having sex with their wives during Affairs Within. I am just saying that you should do something different in these AW games because you are trying to get the juices of love flowing again. You are trying to move in such a way that your bodies and minds can't wait to be together in some secret place that only the two of you know about.

During Affairs Within, you let yourself go. This will require more effort than you normally make in your regular life—more communication, husbands and more sex, wives. Even special things you would not normally do are done in these Affairs Within events. Make your Affairs Within special. Plan them during the year to get you excited for the coming year. Again, it is doing things differently that is the key. If you want something different, you must do something different. There is no other way around it.

Wives should show more flesh (at home especially) during Affairs Within. **So many, many wives look like NUNS and act like NUNS, and in addition tell their husbands they are not getting NONE in the bedroom.** This sort of thing is dealt with by having Affairs Within. Yes, wives, show your husbands what you are working with.

I know you do not as if your stretch marks but let those marks lead your husband down your channel of love. Open up and show it. I am not saying show the world, but you know the clothing that will help give your man a peek every now and then of your body; wear these clothes. Your body belongs to your husband. Husband, your body belongs to your wife.

Your body is not made to be joined up with a harlot but with your mate. There is no other way around this point, so to help ease the process couples must have Affairs Within to ensure that they are keeping the fire burning and allowing their love to pull them in the right direction.

These Affairs Within will allow the husband and wife to be freaks without any inhibitions at all. You will enjoy these times to the fullest. Again, this will involve more sex, but without bickering and complaining. When you schedule your sex times, you should do it no matter what happened that day. You should be totally focused on one another so that nothing comes between you.

When ungodly men and women have affairs, nothing stops them from meeting and having sex on a scheduled day. The same should happen in the marriage as well. You should tell each other that you are on a mission to experience a lot of sex, love, and intimacy, and nothing will stop you.

The powerful thing about having your wife as your mistress is that there are no questions of when you are going to leave your wife because she is your wife. You do not have to pay for two houses or apartments. Those things are already taken care of because you are married to your lover. No second job is needed to pay for the diapers or cloths because you are not the baby's daddy but a father and a husband. There are so many benefits to making your wife your mistress that they completely outweigh the negatives of an external affair.

Affairs Within is not just about sex, but about husbands and wives sharing their dreams without fear of being criticized. During Affairs Within, you will share secrets and desires with each other in order to ensure that you are connected by love. This is the time to keep the marriage engine going and running hot. Men, Affairs Within are not just about you and your penis; they are also about your wife and her brain. Together, you will create a union that is stronger and more cohesive.

Affairs Within should not occur every day; but should happen to prevent the cycle of affairs in the marriage and take the love to an entirely different level. Yes, enjoy your wife as your mistress. Wife, enjoy your husband as the "other man."

In a play written by Bernard Slade called *Same Time, Next Year* (1975),[5] the principal characters are Doris (an Oakland, CA homemaker) and George (a New Jersey accountant). For 24 years, they have an affair one day out of the year at a Northern California inn starting in February 1951. This play was later turned into a 1978 film starring Alan Alda and Ellen Burstyn.

Though George and Doris are married to other people, they continue this romantic tryst without any abandon to the effect of their respective spouses. However, it is funny that they only meet once a year to rekindle their clandestine relationship.

The point I am trying to make is that they carried out this affair for over 24 years. The travel and the lies they had to tell must have been taxing. With six children between them, they went through hell just to meet. To me, George is a perfect example of what a man will do to have an illicit sexual and emotional relationship. If this is true for the illicit, how much more should a husband do for his legal and faithful wife?

George and Doris had to schedule their lovemaking. This point is important. They planned their time together. Even if married couples do not have Affairs Within, it is important to plan the time you will spend together. If you do not plan, you plan to fail.

I know the things I have mentioned in this chapter seem like pipe dreams, but with God in your life and with good communication, you can do it. With many couples, one is trying and the other is not. Such marriages are known to fail.

If you do not have even one Affair Within, then have

many days of forgiveness, mercy, and love toward another. Your marriage vows contain the words "for better or for worse." This may be your worst time as a married couple, but someone within the relationship must be strong and turn the marriage around to ensure an outside affair does not happen. This is not going to happen in a day. It may take weeks or months, but you must try because your marriage is worth it.

References
1. Bader, Michael. <u>Why Men Do Stupid Things: The Psychological Appeal of Prostitutes</u>. 2009. Alter Net. Independent Media Institute.<http://www.alternet.org/sex/79635/why_men_do_stupid_things:_the_psychological_appeal_of_prostitutes/>
2. Dizon, Kristin. <u>Sex Secrets of Escorts: Tips from a Pro</u>. 2005. Alpha publishing.<http://www.seattlepi.com/books/247156_escortsecrets05.html>
3. Alexander,Stephanie. <u>Affairs: Top 10 Reasons Why Men Have Affairs</u>.<http://www.authorsden.com/categories/article_top.asp?catid=44&id=28871>
4. <http://www.wordscapes.net/women-affair.htm>
5. <http://en.wikipedia.org/wiki/Same_Time,_Next_Year>

POWER OF MUTUAL SUBMISSION

Power of Mutual Submission

Ephesians 5 says a couple should submit to one another inside and outside the bedroom. It is very uncommon for couples to love the same thing in the bedroom. Some are lookers and others are adventurous. A couple must find a compromise and submit. If one spouse wants adventure and the other spouse does not, there are going to be problems.

I am telling couples to talk about what they like and do not like in the bedroom. I promise husband and wife you will not go to hell for telling your spouse what you really desire. For some couples it is turtle or hare activity. Whether fast or slow, crazy or conventional, in your marriage you should not hold back. Such actions will cause problems in the end.

Submit may mean try it once in the bedroom. You cannot FORCE anything on each other. Dear Sir, you cannot force your wife to do it. Dear Madame, you cannot force your husband to do it. What I am saying is that you must be open. If it takes years or if you just talk about it, let the conversation begin. Just having a talk about it starts the ball rolling. You are at least opening the door for discussion; you at least give your spouse a talking point.

Submitting in bed is good practice for submitting out of the bed. Once again, this cannot be forced. You cannot beat each other into submission. This includes always asking for the same thing repeatedly. A smart individual will keep the fantasy in her head, and when the time is right, she will lay it on him.

If you never give your spouse what he or she really desires, this spells trouble. When I say desires, I do not mean something totally perverted. Now, the word *perverted* is different for everybody. This is where honest discussion is needed to answer such a question. There must be some type of openness between the couple to discuss these issues.

Even though you may say, "No," today, it does not mean "Never." Together, the two of you can take care of these issues. However, there must be talking and, in talking, you can find answers that will keep both parties happy. Eventually, the talking will turn into action.

I must say, before moving on: If you do not submit, someone will start being unhappy. If you do not give what the other party wants, and it is always YOUR way, then as a couple, you may have problems later. Sex in the bedroom is a journey. It is not just one stop and no more. You have to go beyond the missionary position. It will get boring after a while. Sooner of later, there has to be some spice in the bedroom. If it is nothing but a little bit of pepper or hot sauce, something is needed.

Again, this is about submission. Do not think it should be hot sauce EVERY day. You cannot keep the pedal at 100

M.P.H. all the time. You have to learn how to coast and how to drive fast. There is a need to drive fast and there is a need to drive slowly. You must know the difference. You cannot drive 100 M.P.H. in a 40-m.p.h. zone and vice versa. Some men mess up their groove with their wife because they want her to go fast in a 40-m.p.h. zone, and some women want their husbands to drive slowly in a 100-m.p.h. zone. This is the submission that every couple must follow: find your compromise and enjoy it.

However, men, you should set the first example. You must allow your wife to put out some speed bumps along the way. Men, when you submit to your wife in the bedroom, you plant great seeds. In addition, wives, if your husband submits to your speed, you must submit to his. Without this constant back and forth, you will not be blessed. The marriage will not survive without the constant flow that goes between husband and wife. Without the constant submission, there can be no growth in the marriage. In addition, we all know that if there is no growth, the plant will DIE.

REMOVE THE CHASTITY BELT: OVERCOMING THE GUILT OF FORNICATION AFTER MARRIAGE

Remove the Chastity Belt

We hear that the chastity belt was invented in the Middle Ages to prevent women from having intercourse and masturbation while their Crusading husbands were away—in short, sexual pleasure. Yet, after carefully researching this, I believe that the chastity belt was a metaphor and not something that actually existed in reality.

In any case, we can apply the chastity belt as a metaphor to some dimension of the world we live in. As we look around, we see women bound emotionally and spiritually. To put it simply, something is keeping them from having great sex. This sometimes occurs because of what they learned in their pasts or perhaps their husbands simply do not give them the go-ahead to enjoy sex to the fullest.

In fact, chastity is a good thing for single people. Without a doubt, single people need that metaphoric chastity belt; but once you get married, that belt should be tossed out. Too many times the belt goes back on when one spouse gets mad at the other. You can't continue to do this and expect to be blessed in your union. This cannot and will not last in the long run. Some Christian married couples can't transfer from chastity to sensuality after the marriage ceremony.

Yes, it may be hard because, as singles, we so correctly fought against the flesh and what we wanted to do. But, after marriage, we must fight that stigma and love our spouse to the fullest. When marriage beckons, we need to turn that corner and run to our spouse with open arms and open minds.

Yes, that single Christian person did a great job in keeping holy and pure before marriage. Yet, that person must let go of chastity toward his or her spouse and practice chastity only when it comes to faithfulness. This is where chastity is important: when it relates to faithfulness. Besides that, you are supposed to have great sex with each other without limits or regards. The only limits will be the ones you mutually place on one another as a loving couple.

When you are married and have the mental chastity belt on, it is like going to the amusement park, walking up to the roller coaster, and refusing to get on the ride. You are married now, but you refuse to please one another to the fullest. One person holds back from the other for various reasons. My friends, if you are married, you must enjoy the ride from beginning to the end. You cannot stay cold and expect things to happen on their own.

You must flip the switch and say to one another "It's time to get busy and love each other and enjoy what the Lord has given to us and every couple." If Christian married couples do not take off that chastity belt, shame on them for not enjoying what God has offered them on a silver platter. Shame on them for letting remnants of their single life affect their married life. They must go forward, press on, and get rid of that belt.

For many, this is an ongoing battle between past and

present. A person may be forgiven, but if they do not forgive themselves, all is in vain. This guilt even goes to another level as it relates to marriage; for some, it is like Dr. Jekyll and Minister Hyde. When you were single, you were a freak who went all out for sex, but now that that you are saved and married; you act like a nun or a priest in the bedroom. This explains why many husbands do not like church: their wives turn away from them and become something very different in the bedroom.

Sometimes older people feel they must stop enjoying sex for whatever reason. Get over it! Enjoy your life to the fullest as long as it lasts! Sometimes getting back into lovemaking takes time and forgiveness. God forgives and forgets once we turn to Him. The person who does not let go of the past will carry that scarlet letter wherever they go. Yet the scarlet letter must go. If you are single and converted, you have time until God sends you a mate. You have time to go through the process (letting go of the guilt of fornication) alone, so when the time comes, you are ready to go to the next level with a mate if God permits.

However, if you are married I must be blunt. The process (letting go of guilt after fornication) must go a little faster especially if the husband is not saved. You cannot shut down your womb because you are saved. Such actions will cause the marriage to fail and are ungodly, according to I Corinthians 7. Woman, your body does not belong to you, but to your husband and vice versa. Man, your body belongs to your wife. However, I speak to both men and woman and say all is forgiven under the blood of Christ.

The enemy beats you with guilt when you fornicate as a single person; once you are married, Satan keeps on beating you with that guilt stick. These tricks of the enemy concern your walk with the Lord. You cannot look at this in any other way. The devil wants to keep you bound to him in any fashion that he can, but you must walk in freedom. I understand the past has a funny way of working on you and coming up against you. God knows what you go through and with His help; you will get past your guilt.

Men can easily separate love and sex. Some women cannot. "I love you," to some wives, means, "I want to have sex with you." A wife is expected to show love by having sex. However, resentment and problems in the relationship will occur with this behavior. Sex is an expression of love. The more you demonstrate love, the more you can do things without fear. Husbands must be sensitive when having sex with their wife. Some wives have a fear of being discovered by their own kids while in the act of moving love. However, if you are afraid of being caught, your husband can feel rejected because you refuse to have sex with him.

As I mentioned earlier, past relationships can cause guilt. Sometimes, one spouse carries the baggage of unrealized guilt. This guilt may have been induced by sexual abuse from a father or uncle or neighbor. A little girl or boy can blame herself or himself for the inappropriate and unnatural sex that took place, and the curse is passed on.

It is common for the enemy to try to keep believers from having what God offers to every married believer. God gave married heterosexual couples freedom to have love and orgasms until Jesus comes back. Therefore, in spite of the pains of the past, married couples must fight to embrace each other and their sensual future together

As a cowboy uses the reins to hold back a horse, so sexual guilt from the past holds us back. Whether you are a part of the sex act voluntarily or involuntarily, a person must move beyond sexual guilt. If you do not, then the other spouse will be punished for something that he or she did not do. We have no idea what ghosts and demons hold men and women at bay because of past sexual experiences.

Yet every man and woman must press on and reveal to the spouse all of the problems or experiences. Until you confess what has happened, you will be locked in a cage of guilt and shame.

However, in a way, the other spouse is an escape artist, there to help the guilty one escape. However, you must share this experience with each other. When you are silent, no one can help you. When you are quiet, the demons of the past keep the guilt drum beating in your head. However, when you have another as your coach (spouse), you, with God, have the power to break free from this influence in your life. However, you must fight these things. Just standing there does nothing.

If you do not share your past sexual issues, then your spouse can become a bitter and emotional terrorist as he or she wonders what they did wrong to deserve such treatment. Unbelievably, the person who is there to help can and will turn around and bite you if you do not take care and realize the importance of taking action.

Listen to me loud and clear: if God did not love you, He would have taken away your penis and clitoris when you sinned. That is not the case. You still have it, and it still works. Move now from guilt to freedom in Christ. Not only does Christ make you free in him, not only does he take you from pain to life, but also he can enter your bedroom, minister to you, and set you free.

PROBLEMS WITH SEX

Problems with Sex

Married couples stop having sex for a variety of reasons. They range from personal to outside reasons that help decreased their love for sex. In addition, the majority of those who raise their hands when the subject of not having sex comes up are women because of guilt or outside issues. Most little girls are into relationships with their girl friends while most boys are into sports and sex.

Teenage boys are nothing but a power keg of hormones and a huge goal in life is to procreate at all times. Since this is a fact, this explains why so many men are into sex and have no hang-ups, while girls are a little more reluctant. If you fast-forward 10 or 20 years, you have a grown woman now trying to get her brain around the issues of sex and her husband's desire for her.

One of the biggest problems with sex in a married home is the frequency—how often to do it. This is often a battle between couples, i.e., how much does this person need on a weekly basis? The number can range from one to seven times a week for some men and woman. Hence, this is where the battle starts. Finding the correct answer is

| 127

not easy. Each couple must be honest and open with their needs and desires.

In addition, yes, the Bible does say your body does not belong to you any more, yet there are still elements of sex that can cause trouble for the couple, especially relating to frequency. Your discussion must be done with respect. The spouse less interested in sex must understand that the other one is not nasty or no good; he or she just has a desire to be with you, and thank God for that!

In addition, calling them a dog or other bad names will only hinder the relationship. Each couple must find their own joy. They must find what is needed to get them into the mood to have sex. Once they discover this, the joy must be maintained to keep peace and love in the house. Another issue of sex, premature ejaculation (PE), is a problem for many men. This problem for men only makes the wives less into sex because they see their husbands getting off, but they never share in the fruit of love. Men, the solution to this problem is easy: women first.

Instead of making yourself a priority, let your wife have that power and priority; in other words, make sure she is finished first. Make sure she orgasms first, and then you can orgasm second. Penetration is your last act. Work on her body from head to toe. Touch without being sexual at first. After touching the non-sensual zones, you move on to touch the sensual zones of her body.

While touching her sensual zones, you call attention to the clitoris. Once you have done all that, my brother, now concern yourself with penetration; if the wife so desires at this time. If this pattern is followed every time, more often than not you will have a happy wife in your life. A happy wife is a happy life.

In addition, when the wife is on top, she is in control.

This means easier orgasms for her because she is the one controlling the action. She is the director of the sex movie, and you, sir husband, are the actor.

Some couples have issues about how the penis or the vagina looks. Some people may laugh at this, but it is true in some cases. This can especially happen if sexual abuse happened in the past. The abused spouse will always link the penis or vagina to the past abuse and pain. Thus, they may cause fear in relation to their spouse's sexual organs. There is no easy way of overcoming this. Your spouse is not the guilty party. He was not there during the sexual abuse. In fact, your spouse may have been abused in another way. The point I am trying to make is: do not let the abuser have control over you in your adult life. Sure, pray, but get therapy as well to help deal with your negative images from the past.

As funny as this sound, husbands and wives, your sexual organ is your spouse's friend. They need your organ and you need theirs. In fact, talk about your fears, and never force an apprehensive spouse to do what you desire. Offer love and peace to help the spouse move from bad memories and guilt relating to sexual abuse and fear of the sexual organ.

For others, it is not about abuse, but about being told as a child that sex is dirty and nasty. Of course, this can cause a person to hate everything about sex—even the look of it. Again, talking about one's upbringing will shed light on problems in the relationship. Separately, you were hurt, but together you can bring about solutions that will be great for both husband and wife.

One area seldom discussed involved what I call the 'love towel' or clean up after sex. This may be embarrassing, but fights have broken out over who is going to do clean up duty. One thing I hope married couples will see is that marriage is a partnership. In fact, selfishness cannot enter the picture at all. Therefore, after loving making is done, the person who was pleased the most should volunteer to get the love towel.

This is just an idea for a rule of thumb. When you share in love, you share in work. For some, this is totally out of the question. Some must run to the bathroom and clean up, while other couples cuddle for a while afterward. I have no words for this, but insure both parties are happy with the after effects of sex.

If one party is made to feel dirty and unclean, this might have a psychological effect on the other spouse. If you have learned anything, I hope you have learned that you are trying to take away as many negatives as possible. Do not try to distance yourself from your mate after sex; this is really the time to hold on to each other. However, I know some couples want to do the exact opposite and clean up.

Have an agreement with your spouse on how you are going to deal with the clean up afterwards. Husbands will identify with this fact: if you do not clean up quickly, the sperm will dry and that makes it worse to clean up in the morning. So yes, men, this responsibility may fall on you more often, but the point is not the clean up, the point is the fact that you have to clean up in the first place. Face it, husbands; our goal is to have as many clean ups, as we need in life.

Another factor that affects marriage is sexual positions and different sexual acts. This has been an ongoing debate among church people. As expressed in my other books, *New Sheets* and *Successful Marriages for Successful Men*, I believe the bed is honored in whatever the couple mutually decides to do. I have no commandment for you as to what acts are allowed or not allowed. To me it is very easy: can you give back in the same amount and manner that it was given to you?

In other words, if the husband does it to the wife can the wife do the EXACT same thing to the husband? If the answer is "No," then that sexual act should not be done. For those who say it is nasty or not good at all to have sex in different positions, you are missing the adventure of a lifetime. Find out what you and your wife can and cannot do in the bedroom.

Often, when people are single and dating, their bedroom activities are unlimited, but once they are saved and/or married, they turn off the faucets of adventure. No, my friends. Marriage is the time to turn it on, because when you become a committed married person, not only are you pleased, but also God is pleased because He sees you in a relationship that He and He alone has commanded.

Another quick point: I sometime hear pastors telling couples what they can or cannot do in their own bedroom. What works for that preacher is good for him; maybe he is a control freak and really wants his wife to be a prostitute while he is the pimp. Maybe their role-playing is great. That may work, but what you do or do not do in your bedroom is for you as a couple to decide. It is not necessary for the congregation to know about.

Most importantly, if a couple runs into a no-no that the pastor talked about, and the couple has not yet cleared it with each other, this might bring about finger pointing and pain down the road. This is not good. The Word says to work out your own salvation. I think the same is true for every couple. Couples need to work out the sex in their own marriages. They need to make sure they please one another and NOT the pastor; the pastor is not in bed, the couple is in bed.

Smell and bad hygiene can also disturb sex between spouses. The solution is very clear: wash and keep yourself clean for each other. For some men, the concept of yeast infections is new. They have never heard, seen, or smelled it, but once you get married, it is a common thing. This is not the time, men, to try to persuade your wife to jump in the river, but a time to understand that her body goes through changes and a part of the change is a yeast infection that can come out of nowhere.

In addition, husbands don't realize that after sex with his respective wife, semen left in the vagina cavity takes time to come down. There are times the smell is quite strong and powerful from this residual semen, but remember, she smells that way because of the great sex you had. In these times, have compassion and not distain for your wife. The same goes during her time of the month.

FEARS OF SEX

Fears of Sex

Based on what I see, there are many major forms of fear that deal with sex. Until these fears are overcome, some mates are frozen in their sexual tracks. First, as believers in God, we should not fear, but have faith in God. Fear has no place in the bedroom of a married man and woman. Note all the information below comes from <Wikipedia.com>[1].

Agraphobia or *contreltophobia* refers to fear of sexual abuse. This occurs at times when adults who experienced sexual abuse as children try to deal with the trauma. Any simple move or trigger can carry them back to the place of pain and darkness. According to Wikipedia, this can even occur to those who have watched sexual abuse.

This again opens up reasons why some men or woman cannot enjoy sex. I understood that just having the problem is only half the story. You have to go deeper and discover the trauma and pain you are having within your life and search out the source. As Christians, we all know Satan, as the source of evil, but, again, it is our job to get proper help not only for ourselves but also for those we love.

Erotophobia refers to the fear of sexual love or sexual questions. I believe this is the biggest fear among sexually frustrated Christians. According to *answers.com*[2], erotophobiacs can score high or low on a scale. A low score refers to guilt from sin. These people do not like talking about and feel negatively toward sex, even sex with their spouse. People with high scores are erotophobiacs who have no guilt toward sex and speak openly about it. Yet, sometimes high-scoring erotophobiacs are very open and may be unfaithful to their spouses.

I believe that a low score on the erotophobia scale reflects some Christians who have been instructed incorrectly by ministers who do not really understand scripture. Sex is a great thing; yet, when guilt is placed on it, negative energy will come forth. You cannot just have a prayer meeting in the bedroom; other things must be done.

In other words, Christian couples with fear of sexual love are like caged lions, unable to break free because of fear deep inside them. Everything that God made, including sex, is good. In fact, as I mentioned, the only thing that God called 'not good' was man by himself.

God spoke the words that said man should not be alone. He needed a mate. He needed company. This is the initial reason why God created Eve. He created Eve so that man would not be alone and man could have sex. God created sex for a great reason. . He created it for men and women to share. That is plain and simple; he only placed rules around the boundaries of the marriage. Within the marriage, let the games begin. Let married men and women begin to have sex.

In fact, for some couples, the only way to get this demon out of your bed is to have more sex. Yes, the prescription is to have lots of sex. The more sex you have, the better you will feel and the sooner you will drive away the fear. Talk about the origins of the fear. Find the place it starts, and from there you will begin the healing program within your life. However, the healing must begin and must begin now.

For some, this fear began with a sermon from Mom and Dad that scared them half to death or perhaps it began when a preacher said sex was wrong but forgot to mention that sex in marriage is all right. Oh, we have come a long way. God did not give us the spirit of fear. So if He did not give us fear, why have fear of sex with your spouse? Get over it, and enjoy what God has given you.

Eurotophobia is fear of the female genitalia. This may happen after a wife gives birth because now her husband no longer sees a wife and lover but a mother who has given birth. Therefore, since he would never have sex with his mother, he carries this as if his wife were his mother. In addition, some women do not like how they look sexually. Therefore, if they do not like how they look, they are surely not going to let their husbands look at their genitalia or touch them at all.

Genophobia or *coitophobia*, is the abnormal fear of sexual intercourse. Most of this fear comes from trauma relating to rape or molestation. This is why it is so important to talk about the past as couples begin to think of marriage. A single girl may be a sex freak, but the wife may be a nun because of the pains from her past. So now, a wife has turned from a sex freak to a nun and the husband has no answers.

It is not just knowing that your wife or husband does not like sex; it's asking, "Why not?" This is the drill that every couple must go through to find the solution to problems in marriage. This fear makes it worse, because the offense usually takes place during childhood. This means for all this time the wife or husband has been dealing with a pain that goes all the way back to childhood. This is deep within the self.

How powerful is this fear that grew as the child did. As the child matured, so did the fear; as the child married, so did the fear. This is why prayer and proper treatment are needed to battle such a problem. There is no way this can be done by the individual alone. It needs divine intervention. As with any fear, you must shine light on it. When you have light, there is no darkness or fear in the way.

What I say it is very important because some men hear, for example, from their wives that they were raped or sexually abused. In return, the husband might say, "What's the big deal?" or "No problem." No, you must dive in and understand the domino effect this has on your wife. Some husbands wonder, "What is going on?" When you were dating, this was not the case, BUT now that you are married, the wife shuts down, and you wonder, "What gives?"

This is simple: the fear matures after marriage. At times, even a position or an act can trigger a wife's memory to go back in time. A husband must not turn away but must help his wife in her time of need. This fear can also bring depression because their bodies want sex, but their mind cannot get around it. This is a struggle. This is not the time to run away; this is the time to get proper help to overcome such pain.

Gynophobia is fear or anxiety about being seen naked, and/or about seeing others naked, even in situations where it is socially acceptable. Gynophores may experience their fear of nudity before all people, or only certain people, and may regard their fear as irrational. This phobia often arises from a feeling of inadequacy that their bodies are physically inferior, particularly due to comparison with idealized images portrayed in the media. (answers.com)

These people do not like their bodies. This phobia relates directly to eurotophobia. In all, this will take away from man and woman becoming one. This takes away from what is really needed in the home: comfort and freedom from shame as it relates to your bodies. Again, the origins of this may have started in sexual abuse at a young age. In all, this will affect the husband and wife and the way they interact with one another.

Malaxophobia (Sarmassophobia) is the fear of love play. Put simply, this is a fear of foreplay. In any case, this is not good for the marriage because foreplay is needed in lovemaking. Without foreplay, wives especially, may be limited because most women need foreplay to get things going to reach an orgasm. Without foreplay, you will have no play in the bedroom.

Couples must overcome this with counseling or some other way. When you have such fears, the marriage will be limited in many dimensions and areas of life. Couples must have no limit on what they mutually enjoy doing with each other.

Medomalacuphobia is the fear of losing an erection. This, of course, deals primarily with men who have pre-ejaculation issues; they know they cannot maintain, and so a fear develops. In essence, they give up before they even start. This might occur because a former girl friend spoke with bitterness and pain, or this could happen to a young and inexperienced man who heard stories of men losing an erection. In all, he never tries. He stops before he starts.

On the other hand, some women might have this fear because of experiences where the man they were with before their husband could not keep an erection and this created much apprehension. She may fear that once he has one, it might not last. Yes, I said it. If you are going to have great sex you must last.

There are many ways to battle such issues, but the best one is to talk to each other. It not just seeing the problem; it is knowing that the problem is there and doing something about it. The communication is open and fair to both parties without condemnation. It is not just "Getting over it," it's "Getting over it together."

Medorthophobia is the fear of an erect penis. This is just the opposite of *medomalacuphobia*. This, for sure, comes from abusive experiences. Again, the best way to deal with this is to get proper medical and/or psychological counseling to fight these demons from the past. If you do not fight, the demon will grow inside you. This is why it is so important for the husband to know who his wife is.

Not just sexually, but mentally. In these cases, the erect penis is identified with pain, trauma, and even rape. Therefore, when a woman marries and sees her husband's erect penis, she may automatically have a flash back, which in turn hurts the marriage sexually. This can be overcome, but it takes a willing wife and a patient and loving man.

Oneirogmophobia is the fear of wet dreams or nocturnal emissions. These emissions or ejaculations happen during the night without the man knowingly participating in the act. According to Wikipedia, in the 18th or 19th century men who experienced this often were considered to have the disease *spermatorrhoea*. For some, the cure included castration (the devil is liar) or circumcision. If anything, this proves that ejaculation is a common thing that happens every day to men when there is a build up of semen that must be expelled. There is nothing to fear about this. Yet in the past, many men felt condemnation for having wet dreams, which breeds fear.

According to the Bible (Leviticus 15) , when a man had nocturnal emissions (wet dreams), he had to ceremonial wash. (The same thing applied to women during their period.) Any semen left on the body was considered unclean, and a washing had to take place to take them from unclean to clean. If this is the case, then the sin is not that men ejaculate; the sin is in the cause of the ejaculation. From all I have seen, when you fornicate or commit adultery, ejaculation of semen is wrong. Yet when in a marriage relationship between couples ejaculation of semen is not wrong.

Other forms of sexual fears include: *paraphobia*, fear of sexual perversion; *parthenophobia*, fear of virgins; and sexual aversion, fear of body parts, being touched, and/or sperm.

In all, fear is an enemy to a couple. Fear has no rightful place in the home of a Christian couple. If you are not supposed to fear death, why fear life (sex)? There may be other fears not listed here, but in all, they are fears that married couples must face together and dispel for the glory of the Lord.

Reference:
1. < Wikipedia.com >
2. < http://www.answers.com/topic/erotophobia >

THE MATRIX

The Matrix

The following five scriptures talk about the matrix. Some people do not understand that the matrix did not originate with the movie; the original meaning of *matrix* is the female vagina. All Bible translations are KJV.

Exodus 13:12

That thou shalt set apart unto the LORD all that openeth the matrix and every firstling that cometh of a beast which thou hast; the males shall be the LORD'S.

Exodus 13:15

And it came to pass, when Pharaoh would hardly let us go, that the LORD slew all the firstborn in the land of Egypt, both the firstborn of man, and the firstborn of beast: therefore I sacrifice to the LORD all that openeth the matrix, being males; but all the firstborn of my children I redeem.

Exodus 34:19

All that openeth the matrix is mine; and every firstling among thy cattle, whether ox or sheep, that is male.

Numbers 3:12

And I, behold, I have taken the Levites from among the children of Israel instead of all the firstborn that openeth the matrix among the children of Israel: therefore the Levites shall be mine.

Numbers 18:15

Every thing that openeth the matrix in all flesh, which they bring unto the LORD, whether it be of men or beasts, shall be thine: nevertheless the firstborn of man shalt thou surely redeem, and the firstling of unclean beasts shalt thou redeem.

The word *matrix* in the original Hebrew is *rehem*, which means the womb. Therefore, the matrix is the womb from whence all life emerges. Yet, for centuries, this has been an area of the church world that has been maligned and distorted by priests and pastors alike because they know its power. Instead of trying to understand the matrix, they have preached against its beauty in the marriage arena.

In the Middle Ages, those who decided to get married were considered second-class citizens because they could not abstain from sex. Again, it is simply ignorant to curse and talk badly about something that God gave to every married man and woman. Yet, because people in high places have spoken against the matrix, they have directly or indirectly spoken against women. In fact, women in certain religious circles cannot achieve orgasms because of the condemnation passed down from the ages.

The matrix is not something dangerous in a marriage. In fact, the husband should celebrate what God has given to both him and his wife, but how he cares and loves his wife has a direct impact on the matrix. If the wife is not happy, the matrix will not open. Yet if the wife is happy, the matrix will always be open.

For the wives who read this book, you have the matrix and you should use it for the love of your husband. If you have a faithful and repentant husband who knows he is not perfect but loves you with all his heart, then you need to let him feel the matrix. The Bible says to submit, but it is another thing to submit willingly and lovingly.

I am not saying if your husband is unfaithful you should offer him the matrix, but I am saying if he is loving and caring, you need to give him the matrix. And not just for his enjoyment, but for yours, as well. Because when a man only comes to one place for his needs, it is a powerful thing to any wife. Yes, there are many fast food diners where a man can eat, but when a man only comes to one diner and eats, the owner feels happy and honored.

Well, wives, you should feel the same. Instead of cursing your husband and pouring cold water on him when he comes to you to experience the matrix, you must reward him and hold him to let him know, "Yes, I am happy you have made the decision to make my matrix the only place you go for sexual pleasure and happiness."

Due to the ignorance and bad teachings of the church, some wives and husbands have stopped enjoying the matrix. *Matrix* the movie revealed the behind-the-scenes of true life; I say the same for the married bedroom. Couples must press beyond the mask and venture together into the love and power of the matrix. In the movie, the main character had to press beyond what he saw, as do the wife and husband have to press beyond any inhibitions that stop them from enjoying sex to the fullest. No one, and I mean no one, should control the matrix except for the husband and wife.

When you love your wife, the matrix will love you, but, again, we cannot go beyond something to the next level unless we are ready to live it. When I say live it, I do not mean you must have sex everyday. I mean you always keep it fresh and protected from the outside judgment of people.

The point I am trying to make here is that when couples realize the beauty and power of the matrix, there can be no turning back. You cannot go back to old ways and thinking. You cannot stay where you are; you must press on to stay within the power of the matrix.

I am not saying the matrix is everything, because it is not. God is everything. But, regarding a married couple, yes, the matrix is important. It needs to be respected because the matrix not only brings forth life, it brings forth encouragement. To increase the matrix, you must increase care and communication. Husbands, you cannot expect her to open the matrix if you do not open up and communicate.

Married couples may not have money, but they have sex. Too many times couples focus on what they want and not on what they have already. The matrix is to be shared by the wife to the faithful husband.

Many times, we try to find solutions that are already in front of us. We try to find answers, when the answer is right there. Between communication and the matrix, we have enough to help us during the lean times.

Between good communication and the matrix, during lean times we have something to keep us encouraged and correct when outside forces attack. I am saying, in essence, do not be afraid of the matrix and enjoy what God has given to every married couple.

SARAH'S PLEASURE

Sarah's Pleasure

Sarah, wife of Abraham, was past the age of childbearing when she heard that she would have a child. Upon hearing the message, she said to her husband "How should I have pleasure in my old age?" (Genesis 18:12). The word pleasure in the Hebrew translates as *Eden*. Yes, she said in essence, "How can we have Eden on earth when I am so old?" This confirms my point: the joy and ecstasy of sex between husband and wife is like being in Eden. I believe that sex between a husband and wife is the closest one can get to the Garden of Eden.

Sarah asked the question because her husband was old, too, and she wondered how his member would function again not only for her to conceive but also even for them to start the process. In the end, she had a son called Isaac, but God had to anoint Abraham to bring forth his seed. God had to get involved to make sure Sarah had pleasure—to make sure she delivered a son according to His promise. However, the baby did not come until after she had pleasure. Once she had pleasure, then she had the son. Do you understand the logic?

There is a lesson to be learned by men here, and it is simple. Before you come, let your wife have an orgasm first. See, Sarah did not mind the child, but she also wanted the pleasure. She wanted to feel her husband's love again as she had in the past. She not only wanted the child, but also she wanted the pleasure.

This is not selfish on Sarah's part; she simply wanted to enjoy the ride as well. Too many husbands enjoy the sexual ride while their wives wait at the traffic light on the corner wondering when the bus will come. She ensures her husband's bus. She insures he has an ejaculation, and so it is common sense that she should have fun, too.

Oh, men and women of God, if the mother of the faith (Sarah) wanted pleasure, do not stop until you get what is rightfully yours. Too many women, especially Christians, become mean, bitter old ladies when they withhold themselves from pleasure. I know men can be hard and treat women badly, so that by the time a wife reaches 50 she has retired the matrix.

However, some women out there have good men who have been faithful to the marriage and are reaching old age; do not let that stop you from getting and receiving pleasure from your spouse. It is unbelievable that so many church mothers sit there hurt and broken and desiring the love of their husbands. But, because of so-called church morals, they say, "No," to themselves and indirectly to their husbands.

I rebuke that spirit now. Sarah wanted and GOT pleasure from her husband, Abraham. If Sarah got pleasure, then it is time older wives got their pleasure too. It is time for older married women to break down these fabricated walls and start having great sex again with their mates. Wives, I know you may have issues with vaginal dryness and menopause, but there are products to help you get around these problems so that you can have pleasure.

In fact, (I have absolutely no data for this), the more sex you have, the longer you live. Yes, it is just my opinion, but it makes sense. Orgasms releases so many good hormones that it make since that sex gives good life. However, I think many couples miss the sex and love that God has created for them. Since the vagina and penis do not drop off at a late age, it must mean to keep on using them.

No one told you to give up the "love towel" after a certain length of married life. Keep on having pleasure until the very end. Do not give up on your Eden. I will say it again. Do not give up on your pleasure. It is yours for the taking so take it and enjoy it to the fullest. Do not let man or religion keep you from entering your Eden if you are in a married relationship.

Other words associated with Eden are *delight*, *delicacy*, *living voluptuously*, and *house of pleasure*. Is any one hearing me? Is anyone getting this? We cannot find Eden on a map, but we can sure find Eden in the married bedroom. Since the Bible says there is no marriage in heaven, then we need to get all the loving we can get on earth. Since we are going to heaven, then sex is our Eden on earth. Yes, that is what I said; sex is the Eden that God bestowed on us.

We will NEVER find Eden the place, but we can find Eden the experience. An experience between the married intercourse of a husband and wife.

There are many theories as to what happened to the original Eden in Genesis chapters 1 through 3. The last thing we hear of it is of an angel protecting it so that man and woman would not enter there. However, God in his grace gave us **_another Eden_**. It is between husband and wife and in that passionate moment, we have our Eden back. At one point, Satan led us out of Eden, but at this time we have the opportunity to walk back in and enjoy the moment. We can say to ourselves, "God, I want my Garden back. We want our Eden back."

This Eden is a welcome sanctuary for any married husband and wife; instead of stress, you have the garden. Instead of pain or the problems of life, you have the garden. In addition, as in any garden, the more you work with it, the more results it will return unto you.

To this end, I encourage married couples to stay in the garden and make sure no weeds come up. Make sure no problems negatively affect the Garden. Love the Eden God has given, do not destroy what God gave. For this the revelation comes: God called it good and very good because He gave to those in a marriage relationship a Garden of Eden. We just have to rediscover and nurture it.

As it relates again to Sarah, she saw no limits in pleasure with her husband. Mature wives should take note. The only marriage sexual limits are the ones in the Bible (fornication, adultery, homosexuality, and bestiality) and the ones you set. Supposed limitations are really felt during menopause. Dr. Fulbright says, contrary to popular belief, menopause is a chance to reflect upon and strategize about one's sex life. Often requiring new tricks and sexual experimentation, it can invite some of a couple's most exciting sexual moments. In addition she said, as stated by the National Institute of Health, some women actually feel liberated post-menopause, even reporting an increased interest in sex. This isn't surprising when you consider that once a woman reaches menopause, she (and her partner) don't have to worry about pregnancy, PMS pains or menstruation. The kids are grown and out of the house (hopefully!), so lovers are thrilled that the empty nest has been reclaimed as their love nest. All of these factors can make for more enjoyable, satisfying sex.[1]

In the article, she recognizes the sexual responsiveness of women may be affected by vaginal dryness, less sensation, pain during penetration, pain or soreness post-intercourse, etc. Such things can lead to a lower libido. Yet Dr. Fulbright says by patience, experimenting, communication and a host of other things can break this cycle. The choice again wives are up to you to have pleasure or bitterness in your mature and seasoned years.

Reference:
1. Fulbright, Yvonne K. <u>6 Ways to Boost Your Sex Life After Menopause</u>.2009. FOX NEWS. May 28, 2009. <http://www.foxnews.com/story/0,2933,522658,00.html>

FEMME FATALE

Femme Fatale

Femme fatale, or the sexual prowess of women, has been maligned since the beginning of time. Wives who are in touch with their sexuality have often been ostracized historically by both the religious and secular worlds. For many cultures and beliefs, this has been a constant point of contention for a man who is married to or influenced by a femme fatale. Yet in my opinion, everything that God made was good. The key to this point is a wife should:
1. understand this gift
2. do not use the gift for selfish gain
3. understand that God does not take it away when you become a Christian
4. be under the control of God and use her gift positively
5. understand other men are going to be attracted to her like bees to flowers.

As for the first point, to deny a gift is to waste a gift. Women who are tuned in to their libido have accepted the gift, and this is a great accomplishment. The key is to understand what you have and to enjoy what you have within the confines of married life.

In fact, a wife shares with her husband in order to see her true womanhood to fruition. Womanhood is not just defined by pregnancy, but by knowing every part of your body. A true woman knows how her body functions not only for her own knowledge, but also for the knowledge of her husband and for their lovemaking.

The second point is most important. Once she discovers who and what she is, a woman must not use her gift for selfish gain. No doubt, this gift is not to be used on another man except her husband. <u>If a wife finds out that she has the gift and can control the gift, her options (within the marriage) are boundless</u>. Though this is true, a boundless woman (outside of marriage) is a foolish woman.

A wife who uses her gift of sexuality as an act of revenge or evil is not in any way fulfilling the will of God. For those women who cannot control this, the gift is not deserved. However, wives who use the gift to share with their husbands are golden women who will be called 'blessed,' and their husbands will hurry home everyday. Your job, wife, if you accept it, is to please your husband and in turn, he will please you.

Quick warning husbands, if you are very envious of other men, your wife will not use her skills on you. She will keep her skills to herself and you will loose out in the end. Husbands, she is in your bed so stop with the envy.

The third point: God will not take away your clitoris after you become a Christian. God will not rebuke your erogenous zones once you are baptized. After conversion, a wife will have a closer walk with the Lord, which will only give her the power to use her gift of sexuality in the right form and stage. I have heard of Christian women shutting down their vagina when they get married because they are afraid of offending God when they climax and yell with joy. In turn, this makes an unbelieving man not want his wife to become a Christian because she may shut down her love channel.

Women you are free. You are free to enjoy your body and your husband's body, as well. We cannot forget that in heaven there is no marriage nor is anyone given in marriage there. So, in other words, enjoy it while you can. I have also seen newly Christian wives feel guilty because of past sexual sins. Let me define sexual sins. Any sex between parties outside of marriage is sinful. Therefore, some women come to the marriage with guilt and, of course, this affects the wife and inhibits her fulfilling her needs and taking care of her husband.

Wives must remember that God created all; women did not pick up sensual behavior by accident. No, my sister, God created something good inside of you. In fact, to be theologically correct, the only curse that women received was the pain of childbirth.

Now, follow my logic: if God thought that a sensual woman was sinful and wrong, He would have advocated female castration of the clitoris (**Female** genital cutting (FGC), also known as **female** genital mutilation (FGM)), but He did not. To take it further, God would have ordered male castration of the penis, as well. However, thank God he has not! Therefore, women, enjoy the sensual part of yourself. My point however, is not to let that thing control you, but you control your sensual power within the confines of God's Word and your and your husband's desires.

Point four says that once you discover your sensual side, women, keep your power under the control of God and in mutual respect to your husband. Sex by itself is not evil. Money by itself is not sinful, but the love of money is sinful. So is the love of sex sinful to a point if it goes beyond one's love of God. All of us desire more money. Most couples desire more sex. When that desire gets in the way of God, it becomes a sin within your life. This is something that women must monitor. If they become more engrossed in the sensual and forget the husband, then something will be wrong down the line because now sex has become the creator. Sex is not the creator. Sex is a part of the Creator's work.

Point five is serious and a byproduct of the power of being a sensual wife. The point is that other men will be attracted to you like dogs going after a female in heat. Let me first say a controlled and God-loving sensual wife is not a slut or a whore, she is just in tune with her body and has a desire to fulfill that desire with her husband alone. To any wife who has such a gift let no one call you a name if you remain in the boundaries addressed above?

You may also have to deal with the envy of other women who have not tapped into that side of themselves. Do not let their handicap stop you from loving your husband to the point that he does not know his own name any more. Love him, good wife.

Yet, I digress. Sensual wives must understand that other men will notice such a gift and you must be careful not to use this gift to flirt with other men. Ladies, as you know, it does not take us men long to pick up a signal. You can be in the dark, and, with just one movement, a man will be at your side. Also, wives, if your husband is mad at you and has damaged your self-esteem, do not find another man to build it up.

If you do so, then you use your gift wrongly, and you

become a woman of the night. I know this sensual side of you can be a burden, but it must be understood and constantly regulated with respect to your husband.

In understanding all the above five points, women will ensure their enjoyment without going overboard. For men, the simple point is to understand the power of your wife's sexual strength and not deny the multiorgasmic character that is within her. From antiquity, men have been envious of women's ability to reach multiple orgasms. For most men, the refractory period—the time it takes a man to reload to launch sperm—gets longer as they get older. A woman, on the other hand, can have WAVES of climaxes, while the man can only have one at a time. Some men, of course, are different, but most men follow this norm of one hit at a time.

Men, do not be jealous of your wife if she is multiorgasmic and sensual. As long as she is not hitting on other men, what is your problem, my brother? You have to grow up and let your wife enjoy her God-given talents. In passing, husbands, the fact that you make such good love that your wife is multiorgasmic and may have additional fluids coming out of her is a compliment to your lovemaking skills. My brother, the more she sweats, yells, and desires more from you sexually, what is your problem? As long as she is not using sex to derail or avoid conversation what is your problem? Enjoy the ecstasy!

We are Christians, not Muslims. The strict orthodox Muslim faith covers everything on women from head to toe because Muslim men do not want their women out in the open. Christian men may do this covering up their wives from a mental point of view. Men, this is not wise. When you hold back your wife, she will hold you back. Let me be blunt. Would you rather she experiences a climax with you or with a stranger? I think, husband, you want to be in the driver's seat.

Your wife will love you for putting aside your pride and for helping her in achieve her climax. For a wife to be free, you must set her free from the genie's bottle that culture and religion have put her in. Husbands set your wife free and she will turn you free in the end. One ingredient to doing this is not looking at your wife negatively or as an ungodly femme fatale.

The very definition of a femme fatale is a woman of great seductive charm who leads men into compromising or dangerous situations (from the French, for fatal woman). There are surely such femme fatales out there. Yet a Christian wife should not feel related to them. She should see herself as using her seductive charm to please her husband and using her charm to excite the Christian bedroom.

The double standard is well in place our society. Men are allowed and encouraged to be charming. Ever heard of Prince Charming? Yet a wife who uses her charm to please her husband is looked upon by some as being a slut. No, she is not a slut if she uses her charm to please her husband. A wife must feel comfortable. When a wife really lets go and abandons her inhibitions, a husband must be able to handle this side of her. For some men, seeing the wife wanting sex as he does makes him nervous. A man may even call his wife a 'dyke' or a 'femme fatale,' but such assessments are wrong.

She is only letting go what has been inside of her for the longest time. Our job as husbands is to allow our wives to find and enjoy the sensual side without condemnation. If a wife is condemned, she may start to charm using a hidden agenda and sexual allure to get what she wants.

Any smart man will want to please his wife and meet her needs. <u>However, a smart man will let his wife use her charm to get something out of him that he was going to give her already</u>!

When a good asset is constantly abused, it may turn into a bad one. A wife who has been beaten down for being sexual may become negative and or a femme fatale. For some people, the church, again, has capped something that really only needed the control and mutual respect of God and husband. It is one thing to <u>control</u> sensuality; it is another thing to <u>destroy</u> sensuality. Churches, through the ages, have tried to destroy the sensual side of women, yet, because women knew it would come back, they became angry and sometimes played the negative femme fatale.

In Genesis 38, Tamar had to play the role of a femme fatale because Judah would not honor his oath to give her to his youngest son (Shelah in Genesis 38:11). Yet, because he did not honor his promise, she had to play this role to give birth to the future king of Israel (David, in generations to come). This is where wisdom comes into play with a wife as it relates to the husband.

In no way am I advocating going outside the relationship, but, in this case, Tamar had to use her charms to fulfill a prophecy. Wives, the power of your charm can make a husband move when he does not want to move. Your charm will make him leap tall buildings in a single jump. This is what charm can do when used with the right motives as approved by God.

Tamar was in a *levirate* marriage. For a male, this was the practice of marrying the widow of one's childless brother to maintain his line, as required[1]. The widow was supposed to be honored. Judah was the so-called protector until his youngest son grew up. But, Judah did not protect. Because Judah did not protect her, Tamar had to protect herself with her own God-given talents. Judah's sons did not pick Tamar, but Judah did. It was an arranged marriage. Nowhere do you see Tamar being whorish or acting out of line as long as the man kept the covenant. As soon as promises were broken, her femme fatale instincts took over.

The lesson learned is for wives to watch their actions when their husbands do not maintain their promises and for husbands to ensure they monitor and keep their promises. When a husband does not keep his word, problems are just waiting to come up and bite the couple.

On the other hand, Tamar used her gift not to get BACK at Judah, but to help him keep a promise he made that he broke. (Again, I am not advocating that wives use their bodies solely to get things out of their husbands. However, you have a power within you; with wisdom you can push the right buttons to get things accomplished.) <u>Remember: It is one thing to beat a man down for not his keeping promise. It is another thing when a wife uses her charm to cause the fulfillment of a promise</u>.

Tamar's name in Hebrew means *palm trees*. She could have used her charm to torch Judah, but she used it instead to fulfill a promise and in the process bring shade to the situation. Tamar had every right to seek revenge, but instead she kept it in the bloodline. She remained in the family to keep the promise alive.

In fact, nowhere in scripture is she rebuked for her ruse. No one puts her down because she was after a promise. She is even mentioned in the genealogy of Christ our Lord (Matthew 1:3; Thamar is really Tamar). <u>Wives, hear me. Tamar teaches you to use your charm not to harm but to get your husband to fulfill his promise</u>. If your husband has broken promises, then use the power of your charm and sensuality to get him to fulfill the promise. Instead of arguing or fussing, use your God-given charm, wives.

I hate to go here, but Eve used her charm on Adam to do wrong. God gave charm to you wives for good or evil. Yes, that decision rests with you. You can use charm to build a man up or use your arguing to bring a man down to the ground.

I think we may have hit upon the reason for the use of charm; it is to get promises from your mate fulfilled. In *Spirit of the Reformation Bible*[6], we see that Tamar met trickery with trickery. Today, wives must ensure they do not use their gift for trickery; rather they should use their charm, their clothes, and their bodies to get a husband to fulfill a promise. Fulfilling a promise does not have to be sexually related. It could just be, "Honey, you promised to go to the doctor for your annual checkup." This is a small example, but if a wife dresses nicely and applies the charm, that man will go to the doctor everyday.

Because of her actions in Genesis 38:26, even Judah calls Tamar's actions righteous. What a conclusion! The righteous man calls the woman righteous for his unrighteous act. We learned that charm, if applied well and controlled by God, is righteous. A wife will not be called femme fatale but righteous, for her wisdom and knowledge.

Theologians cannot deny that Tamar dressed like a harlot. Ladies, I think you know where I am going with this last statement. She dressed to get her father-in-law's attention. I say you dress to get your husband's attention. Whether for pleasure or for sex, a wife, as well as a husband, should always dress to impress. Too many times that is not the case. Some couples dress to repel, especially in bed. Such actions should not take place.

You dress well because you should dress well. Please. I am not saying revert to exhibitionism. But women should dress as a good femme fatale for her husband. She plays the role to have her and their promises fulfilled. There is so much in this area of playing the game. She could have taken her game outside the family, but she kept the game within.

Women, when you take your femme fatale outside, you commit adultery; but when you use you charm within the bounds of marriage, you are a wise and blessed person. Again, please hear me. I am <u>not</u> saying, "Wives, use your charm for evil or harm." I say, "Use your gift to reach God-given promises." Is not a marriage a God-given promise? Then, a wife is correct to ensure that her husband keeps promises made before God and herself. In addition, even when they are kept, she uses her charm and sensuality to reward the man for his faithfulness. A Biblical wife will use her charm to encourage, not bring down, her mate.

Two other women who could be considered femmes fatales are Leah and Rachel. These two Old Testament wives went after Jacob with out abandon. They not only threw their bodies at Jacob, but they threw their handmaids as well. By the time the dust had cleared, Jacob had produced 13 children from four different women. The two handmaids were dowry from Laban, father of Leah and Rachel.

This all happened because Jacob failed to show love to his first wife. Because Jacob loved his second wife Rachel more, his first wife Leah gave him more babies to help Jacob see the love she had for him. Because Leah produced so many babies, Rachel gave her handmaiden (Bilhah) to Jacob; Rachel at this time could not produce children. When Leah saw this move, she gave her handmaiden (Zilpah) to

Jacob. The name Bilhah in the Hebrew means *timid*. She would become the mother of Dan and Naphtali.

In antiquity, for Jewish women, not producing a son or being barren was a sign of a curse on the wife. Rachel wanted to help God by giving Bilhah to her husband. In the end, even though Bilhah gave two sons to Jacob, Reuben (Jacobs' oldest son) had a sexual relationship with her. This, again, shows how the arrangement really did not work out.

Reuben, because of this disrespect to his father's bedroom, lost his birthright. (I guarantee you; the sex on that night of passion was not worth losing his birthright!) In fact, Reuben's birthright, or the glory of the father, was given to the sons of Joseph. Zilpah, the other handmaid, was another tool of Jacob. She had two sons called Gad and Asher.

In those times, handmaids were the property of the women, not the men. This is why Zilpah obeyed without hesitation. In this pattern, the women used their sex appeal to compete, instead of using their appeal to have Jacob love them for who they were.

Here is a decisive test to see if a wife is becoming a femme fatale: assess her motives. In other words, is she using her charm to get the man to love her for whom she is? For Leah, after the third child, she just did the things to encourage herself. The ego works in women as well as men.

Women, always investigate your motives when you use your charm. Some women, at the other extreme, feel no need at all to use their charm on their husbands. It is as if the woman, once married, removes the charm gene and places it in a shoebox. No. Wives take out the charm and use it to the maximum on your husband. Charm has been beaten; but charm used on your husband is a great thing. Delilah used her charm on Samson, why cannot a wife do the same for good motives on a husband?

It seems some Christian women have just put away the pleasure of charming their husbands. Now, I understand a man's attitude can change, and the duration of a marriage can affect a wife's feeling for her husband. But I submit, if there is no adultery involved, if the wife charms her husband—once the husband treats her as nicely as he did when he first meet her—I bet that man would love his wife to charm him. The highway of love works both ways.

Along with Rachael and Leah, we have also Delilah, Salome, Jezebel, and the list of Biblical women who used their bodies for specific gains goes on. Salome used her talents to kill John the Baptist at the request of her mother, Herodias. In fact, it really was not Salome who thought of it, it was her mother who gave Salome the instructions (Mark 6:21-23 & Matthew 14:6).

The account goes like this: Herod Antipas wanted Salome (his stepdaughter) to dance for his birthday. The celebration of birthdays originated in Greece and Rome and not in Jewish custom. So in essence, he should not have participated in it, but he did. In addition, his wife (Herodias), whom he stole from his brother Herod, the tetrarch Philip, gave her daughter (Salome) for his celebration.

Many theologians feel that Herod Antipas' feelings for Salome went beyond those of a father for his daughter. For all we know, this could have been a recorded pedophilia moment: the man who could not get off with his wife instead lusted after his daughter. The mother of Salome sacrificed her daughter for her own good. This poor child was so messed up, she married her father's half-brother Philip the tetrarch, later. Salome danced the Dance of the

Seven Veils in such a way that Herod Antipas wanted to give her half his kingdom.

There is a lesson to be learned by a wife who has a faithful husband. **There is no limit to the love a husband will show for a wife that pleases him.** Even though the circumstances around John the Baptist were not righteous, there are points to be understood from them. I think Christian wives see the work of those who are not saved and shun everything that they do.

I propose that, as Christians, we learn from the world; we still use the inventions of sinners every day. Why not learn points we can possibly apply in our bedrooms? Overall, there are many deadly things to eat in the world, but if the things are cooked well or another element is added to the poison, the poison turns harmless.

Christian wives, Salome's motives were wrong, but if placed in the right situation, her charms would have made another man happy.

What I am saying is that Christian wives who have godly principles should not feel condemned when they use their charm for good or sensual pleasure toward their husbands.

Herod Antipas ruled Galilee and Perea as tetrarch, 4 BC–39 AD. I mention his reign to point out that his rule might have been longer if he had had a smart wife, and not a femme fatale, in his life. Though a man is responsible for his actions in the end, a wife can encourage or discourage a man from doing the right or wrong thing—ask Adam. Again, the final decision is the man's, but a wife can help move the couple over a cliff or into paradise. Instead of using her charm to get her needs met she could have used her charm to encourage and give him wisdom.

It is said and it is true that men are hard of hearing

when it comes to taking suggestions from their wives. Yet, I propose, if a wife uses her charm every now and then instead of her anger, things might be a little different around the home. Some women offer only discouragement and never a word of encouragement. However, ultimately, if a man does his best, his wife will perform her best as well. These are just some things to ponder and keep in mind.

Moving from the religious, there have been many secular femme fatales. Men in general do not want a woman who is comfortable with her own sexuality. Some men fear that their wives will end up like *Mulher Sentada*, a woman in the 1916 painting by Austrian painter Gustav Klimt. (*Mulher Sentada* painting is considered a femme fatale because it depicts a woman pleasuring herself).

Yet in this section again, I encourage men to allow their wives to be whom and what they are. Let me ask you men, if your wife can trust you with your body, why cannot you trust her with her own body? I know this is a scary thing for men, but we must allow women to be free to express their sexuality to us without apprehension.

Chinese mythology discusses concubines and how they brought on the downfall of great men by seducing men to neglect their duties[2]. Yet, the opposite can be done as well. In fact, a wife can use her skills to help a man keep his skills, meet his duties, and reach for greater things in life. Again, if you do not know the purpose of your gift, you will use it wrongly.

I say to wives, use your charm to lift your husband to the next level. A wife can use her ways to help a man when he is down. A wife can do things to her husband that no other can do to tell him to keep up in the race. Therefore, men, do not discourage the power of your wife's sensuality because, in knowing her sensuality, she is able to charm you when you cannot get up on your own.

One famous, real-life femme fatale was Mata Hari who, around the early 1900s, was a successful courtesan known for her sensuality and eroticism rather than for her striking classical beauty[3]. For her role as a so-called double spy, she was executed by the French government for using her charm in the wrong manner on October 15, 1917, at the age of 41.

Another femme fatale in Hebrew folk lore includes Lilith. According to the folk lore, she was the first wife of Adam. Because she refused her husband's sexuality, she was banished from the garden and god (god in small letters because I believe this is only folklore) had to create Eve. Lilith is looked on as representing female empowerment[4]. In all, she is to be feared because she is dangerous, especially when she does not get her way. (See this story of Hebrew folk lore in the *Alphabet of Ben Sira*.)

In most films, the femme fatale uses her power to gain independence and to manipulate men. Overall, *noir films* (dark and brooding movies suggestive of danger); portray the femme fatale as directly attacking traditional womanhood and the nuclear family[5].

I am suggesting just the opposite. In films, the femme fatale controls her own sexuality outside of the marriage. I suggest a wife control her sexuality within the marriage and not outside it. Again, the secular world has portrayed unfaithful women as only having great sex outside the marriage; this means only orgasms with strange men.

I say great orgasms happen within the marriage and not outside of it. The church, though, has discouraged such freedom for women for centuries. I say there is freedom for wives and it's with their husbands. They relish their freedom by staying with their husbands and finding fulfillment in his loins and not the loins of an adulterer. In other words, husbands, release your wife within her sexuality. As long as the sex is coming your way, all is well.

Reference:
1. < http://www.answers.com/topic/levirate>
2. <http://www.answers.com/topic/femme-fatale>
3. <http://www.answers.com/topic/mata-hari >
4. <http://www.answers.com/topic/lilith>
5. <www.lib.berkeley.edu/MRC/noir/np05ff>
6. <u>Spirit of the Reformation Study Bible: New International Version (NIV)</u>, Zondervan .2003

TORI AMOS: THE VOICE OF A GENERATION

Tori Amos: The Voice of a Generation

Tori Amos is a very talented young woman who writes secular songs. However, what make her so special is that she grew up in a Christian home. She had a demanding Christian father, and she has said that his hard convictions affected her sexuality.

Christian children know that they did not get here by a plane or by birds and bees. Yet many Christian parents are quiet on this subject, or they are just the other extreme and do not allow their children to even have air as it relates to talking about sex and its use in the proper perspective. Tori Amos had such an upbringing and is now a popular critic of Christianity, especially in the arena of sexuality.

I believe Amos desires a walk with God but she also wants her sexuality. I say this task can be accomplished within the right boundaries. However, I believe these boundaries are learned as a child. When Christian children are not taught the word of God as it relates to sex, they become either timid or wild in their understanding of sex. Most Christian women are in this ballpark of trying to reconcile this. Amos is not alone in this quest for holiness <u>and</u> sensuality.

Tori Amos is the third child of Rev. Dr. Edison and Mary Ellen Amos, of North Carolina. In their home, they did everything strictly by the book. She began her journey in this stifling, suffocating environment with no air. To add to her tragedy, she was raped as a young adult in California. Her rape affected her, of course, and she wrote a song about it called "Me and a Gun." She is known for emotionally intense songs that cover a wide range of subjects including sexuality, religion and personal tragedy. The rape also inspired her to start RAINN (Rape Abuse and Incest National Network), a toll-free help line in the U.S. connecting callers with their local rape crisis center.

Some women find it hard to admit that they have been raped by their own husbands. When I say 'raped,' I mean forced to have sex that was not enjoyable at all. Men, on one hand, do not understand that, as it relates to sex, women are emotional creatures that MUST have their hearts and minds into the sexual dance. This is why if sex is explained at an earlier age, a woman can gauge her sexuality instead of finding it out totally by herself. Sex is like a bomb. If you do not know how to take it apart or touch it properly, the bomb will go off. This is what happened to Tori Amos and countless other women whose first time was an exploding bomb of a nightmare.

Many men have no clue and never even ask their spouse, "What was your first time like?" Many men would be surprised to find out that the first time was not one to write home about. In fact, the first and subsequent times may have been downright rape. When husbands ask their wives about their sexual pasts, they find they have a lot to learn. <u>The more you know about your wife's sexual history</u>

(without getting jealous), men, the more you can minister to her.

I believe most women need a healing sexuality. Often, sexuality was not explained to the fullest, and because of that, the true definition of this act is never discovered. And if it is discovered, no one explains how this thing works. In fact, most women in their 20s do not reach their sexual prime.

According to Dr. Laura Berman she says" While Planned Parenthood says that the sexual prime for males is around age 17, and that females' sexual prime is around age 30, these ages actually reflect the genital prime, when sex hormones (testosterone in men; estrogen in women) are highest. But in general, both men's and women's sexual performance will peak when they feel most comfortable with themselves and their sexuality. Though this tends to happen between 40 and 60 for both men and women, it can really happen at any age, depending on the person!"[1]

On the other hand, boys have orgasms as soon as they have wet dreams.

So when a husband adds a negative to his wife's sex life, he has more to deal with down the road. He wonders why she does not let herself go sexually. He wonders why the love and power is not there. The simple answer is because there is no room for such. There are too many bad memories that hold the wife to a certain point from which she cannot be released. The wife is dealing with her demons, and she cannot come forth.

I believe Tori Amos MAY be dealing with this demon. But she is not alone. Many girls raised in Christian homes wrestle with this same type of issue and, husbands, it's your job, through God, to settle this issue and show them the light of godly sexual relations. To say the least, Amos speaks her mind. She speaks of personal tragedy that includes the death of brother and baby, yet she continues. Not in a Christian pursuit, but in her own way. When it comes to sexuality, she is straight up and gives it to you like it is, including her opinions and reflections. Once Amos grew up, all of those issues were released as an adult.

This is not the coming-out party that many Christian women have not had, nor do they understand their own sexuality and truly enjoy sex with their spouse without condemnation. Too many Christian women go to bed wanting more but getting nothing because of the way they were raised. Some women in the church used to be in the world; now they are saved and want to run from all sex—even sex in their marriage because they are trying to exercise the demons of their wild nights. This is a fact, and it occurs daily. I look at Tori Amos as a young woman who had to discover her sexuality the hard way to which she is direct and does not care who listens to her about her sexual freedom.

Ladies, I am not saying to go out and buy sexual aids, take them to church, tell the world you are sexually free and you are giving your husband the best sex of his life. I am only saying to wives as it relates to your bedroom you are free.

When Christ died, rose and ascended, it was freedom not just from sin, but freedom from others that binds you or holds you back from experiencing all God has for you. When one holds back the blessing of God, one also is limited in that field. Wives, free yourself sexually.

Tori Amos wrote:

I grew up in dirt-poor hillbilly country. We lived this dry-below-the-waist kind of scene. If you were a sensual woman, you were in league with that which is un-Christ like. Where I come from, a cockroach is a roach, and a cockerel is a rooster because they cannot bring themselves to say c??k.[2]

We may laugh at her comment, but such is the case in many homes. Because of misinformation of the church, the word c??k cannot be spoken. I realize it is a slang word for penis; such ideas can affect a little girl for a lifetime. Not really understanding her libido and the male body parts can have strong and powerful reflections down the road. Though I do not agree with much of what Amos does and says, she is right that a sensual woman is looked on as un-Christ like. The point is, if a young woman is in a marriage, there is nothing with her wanting to experience sex to the fullest with her husband.

The church in some circles is in the Dark Ages as it relates to sex. Some pastors are afraid of the word and action, but such thinking will only produce more young women like Tori Amos. So, how do we move on from this period to another period in our lives? We must be Bible based, but we must set people free so that they have the blessing that God allows all to see and feel within a heterosexual marriage.

The following is a small portion of an interview that Tori Amos had with *Rolling Stone* magazine:

Interviewer: Are some of the same themes appearing— especially concerning female sexuality and religion?

Tori Amos: It was very conscious with [2002's] *"Scarlet's Walk"* and *"The Beekeeper"* that I wanted to embody the Mother Maiden and core essences within the being— because I find a lot of women, especially in this time of the right wing, don't know how to be spiritual and sexual. Either they are puritanical, or their (breast) are hanging out all the time— that has been a real bee in my bonnet, the program that [tells women] to be sexual. To [counter] that, you have to be nasty. I grenade that idea right out of the water!

One side of you might be that vulgar tart, and I will hang out with her. I do not mind a dirty girl. However, what I find tragic is when we, as women, become not the subject of our own story but someone else's object. That, to me, is playing into this role that women have held in Christianity for a long, long time. I refuse to be victimized by Christianity's misrepresentation of our great mothers. I want to be an integrated woman.[3]

Again, this singer who has sold over 12 million albums is direct, but her point of being victimized is true. I do not agree with all of her beliefs about Christianity but I do believe she has it right about the wife's sexuality being controlled by the church.

Through the ages wives have been rebuked and abused for what God has given them. Change must take place to free women of this slavery.

Once a wife has taken authority over her body, she then places that authority in her husband, just as the husband gives the authority of his body to his wife. Together, they form a powerful bond. Yet women cannot give what they do not possess. There is no way a man can move on or a woman can move on if both parties do not have control of what they possess.

Wives posses your assets in conjunction with your husband. Do not be ashamed of what the Lord has given you. You should not be ashamed of your walk with God; you should not be ashamed who you are sexually.

References
1. Dr. Laura Berman. Challenge Your Sex

Preconceptions <http://www.everydayhealth.com/sexual-health/101/tips/challenge-your-sex-preconceptions.aspx>
2. <http://en.wikipedia.org/wiki/Tori_Amos >
3. Robertson, Jessica. Q&A: Tori Amos Talks in Tongues. 2006. Rolling Stone. 30 Mar. 2006 <http://www.rollingstone.com/news/story/9549653/tori_amos_talks_in_tongues>

VICTORIAN MORALITY

Victorian Morality

Without a doubt, our society was shaped by the views of the Victorian period. In short, the views were reserved and allowed a husband's enjoyment of sex but not the wife's. Don't get me wrong, there are good things that came out of the Victorian period as it relates to sex, but there were some beholding things, as well, that have, for the most part, hurt wives across this nation.

The Victorian period can be associated with uptight and self-righteous beliefs and attitudes toward others. Again, there is a need for this as it relates to singles, because of the holiness of God. However, there is a loving platform that I believe God gives to married heterosexual persons that is not mentioned or practiced within this period. Again, the morality of the Victorian period is truly needed for unmarried couples, but as it relates to marriage, all bets are off.

The Victorian period, named after Queen Victoria of England, who reigned from 1837 to 1901, affected the known world strongly because of the power of the British Empire at the time. Yet, with all their standards, there was an understandable hypocrisy going on.

Men were getting their sexual needs met, but women were in the dark sexually. I am just pointing out that when it comes to sex, in the church, many of us have been taught through osmosis or direct preaching that married couples should not enjoy it.

In fact, married Christian couples should have great and loud sex because it was given to us, not only to procreate, but also to bring pleasure to one other and to God. As discussed earlier, the only bad thing that God saw was man being alone. He said that was not good. Yet married men and women who had good intentions in the Victorian period failed to let the freedom flow.

Understanding the background of Queen Victoria is very important to understand her era. In 1840, she married her first cousin, whom she loved dearly. When he died at 42, (December 14, 1861) it totally messed her up to the point that she wore black for the rest of her life and never remarried. In fact, the last thing she wanted her subjects to think about was sex; and, thus, we have unspoken rules for thinking about sex that affect our world even to this day.

I believe this is important because I think we are still fighting the Victorian laws as they relate to marriage. The unspoken laws meant the missionary position and no enjoyment of sex; but this is not the will of God. Furthermore, when you follow such restrictive rules, you raise the risk of rebelling or going against the laws of God.

In essence, the Victorian age that we Americans see today has caged many married couples to the point they do not feel at liberty to express themselves sexually within their home. I hope, through this book, we can let these things go and fully enjoy the plate that God has set before married couples.

Queen Victoria loved her husband so much that she went into self-exile from the public for three years upon his death. Some historians believe that she may have even tried to contact him from the dead through spiritualism. In all, Queen Victoria's pain was transferred to the era that we know today.

I believe that she inserted into our society her grieving as well and a belief that married couples should not have great sex. Most people do not know that she had nine children, which tells me she did have sex with Albert. Once he died, however, it appears she wanted to stop all the pleasure that she could not feel anymore. A quote attributed to Queen Victoria says, A marriage is no amusement but a solemn act, and generally a sad one (answers.com). If she truly said this, it certainly explains her frame of mind toward marriage.

In fact, singles and unsaved persons have enjoyed and even loved sex, but it is seem like married couples have lived in the Stone Age when it comes to loving. I come with this book to set husbands and wives free.

Despite her claims to no longer enjoy passion, rumors abounded that Queen Victoria had an affair with John Brown, a Scotsman and her personal servant. She is known to have given him medals, paintings, and other elaborate gifts.

When sex did come to the forefront during Victoria's reign, it came in 1888, in the form of Jack the Ripper, London's infamous killer of prostitutes. In many ways, this figure, which was never caught, captured the attention of London and the entire country. The message it sent. ONLY ungodly men and woman have wild sex. This is not the case. Wild and great sex is for committed married couples. Couples can have great sex by staying within the boundaries that they both agree upon.

As it relates to morality, the Victorian era is known for its fight against prostitution, the great social evil that prospered in Britain. Without a doubt, this grew out of the problem of many single women and not enough men to go around. This remains an issue today. Some men would rather be johns than men of their own home. Yet, the woman in the street is no different from the wife at home; with the exception of the assumed freedom that a woman in the street has over some wives at home.

I submit again: if wives and husbands felt the same freedom as prostitutes do in making love, I believe the whole institution would go away. I will restate it: if husbands and wives were free with one another in the bedroom, their would be no need of prostitution.

To combat prostitution, the great evil of Britain, in the 1800s the Victorians stressed the importance of female purity and homemaking, with which I agree. However, again, some wives and husbands have taken the purity thing to a point that they no longer enjoy sex and sex is a dirty word.

Because they wanted to get rid of prostitution in their era, they may also have killed the sexual practices of married couples. In short, couples were told to be pure and clean in the bedroom; men may have said to themselves subconsciously, "If I really want to enjoy sex, I must go outside the home." However, what I want to tell men is that they can enjoy sex within the home, and they do not need to creep outside of it.

During the Victoria era, purity was stressed for wives, but not for husbands. This created a double standard that lingers even to this day today. If the wife has to be faithful, so does the husband.

Also influencing Queen Victoria was her uncle George IV, whom she saw as a playboy[4]. When Queen Victoria assumed power, she wanted to rid the monarchy of sandal and pain. (However, there was more talk of this than action. Sunbathing was discouraged as lewd behavior, yet Queen Victoria drew and collected nude male drawings.)

Women's fashion did not permit any show of skin, undergarments or stockings, and cosmetics were forbidden. The point being to be unattractive toward the opposite sex. Now, some wives have taken this to the point of not even doing this for their husbands. I believe a wife should not advertise to the world, but they should look good for their husbands. The Victorian age suffocated the minds of wives, and the husbands went to prostitutes for what they wanted to see.

It was even seen as acceptable for men to have sex with slaves or prostitutes because they were unequal or below the proper man (*answers.com <Victorian women>*). The key is that there were ways of getting around this issue. The other side to this is that the men were given a pass, but woman were not. The same restrictions sometimes exist today, with it okay for men to be the sexually wild one, but the wife has to be the quiet one.

During the Victorian era, parents tried to deal with masturbation from this strict perspective; they even went so far as to deal with the issue using anti-masturbation devices for children (*"Sexuality & Modernity: Victorian Sexuality"*, *<www.isis.aust.com>*). During the age, masturbation was called "solitary vice" or "onanism."

The main reason why Victorians attacked masturbation was because it went against the main premise: sex for procreation only. No procreation, no sex. This was a key point in the Victorian Age. Without the results (babies), the Victorian age saw no need for sex at all (officially, of course). With this in mind, orgasms and climax NEVER entered the minds of married women. In fact, though, the man's needs were to be met, while the wife's needs simply did not exist (officially).

For most men, orgasms and ejaculation seem the same but they are not. These are two different things in both sexes, but for a woman, it takes a while to achieve. Therefore, the Victorian age allowed enjoyment for men, but not for the wife. Once again, the husband was able to "get off," but the wife was restricted.

During this era, Jean-Martin Charcot[1] started his studies on hysteria, which was really a woman having an orgasm, and "man" considered it a sickness. Funny how men during this area had no problem with their hysteria, but when woman had their hysteria, they were looked at as sick. However, Dr. Charcot classified these actions as a disorder in women—a disorder because wives were not supposed to enjoy sex. This was only for the husband, but the devil is a liar. Again, men were to enjoy it while women were supposed to simply supply their husband a receptacle.

Working with Charcot was Sigmund Freud. Even though I disagree with many of his points, he did bring sexuality into the social arena. Jennifer Morley, in her article, "The Victorian Sexual Double Standard in Jane Eyre," says, "Women were expected to show voluntary restraint from the act of sex and shrink from the pleasures of passion."[2] Yet men during this period had sex like rabbits while the wives were supposed to remain chaste.

Without a doubt, the Victorian age affected much of what we do today. In addition, as uptight and hypocritical as the Victorian age was, there is not much difference in our age. In Michael Mason's book, *The Making of Victorian Sexuality* (1995), this point is made perfectly clear. "Despite all of their high standards, people were yet doing things behind closed doors for their own satisfaction."[3]

We thank God for the Victorian Age; it was an age that taught purity in which singles could learn. However, as it relates to couples, it has repressed many attitudes toward sex. In Christ, there is liberty, and, yes, this extends to the bedroom of every married heterosexual couple.

Reference
1. <http://en.wikipedia.org/wiki/Jean Martin_Charcot>
2. Morley, Jennifer. The Victorian Sexual Double Standard in Jane Eyre <http://www.umd.umich.edu/casl/hum/eng/classes/434/charweb/morley1.htm>
3. Mason, Michael. The Making of Victorian sexuality. New York: Oxford University Press. 1995
4. <http://www.answers.com/topic/queen-victoria>

CHURCH ATTITUDES ON SEX FROM ANTIQUITY

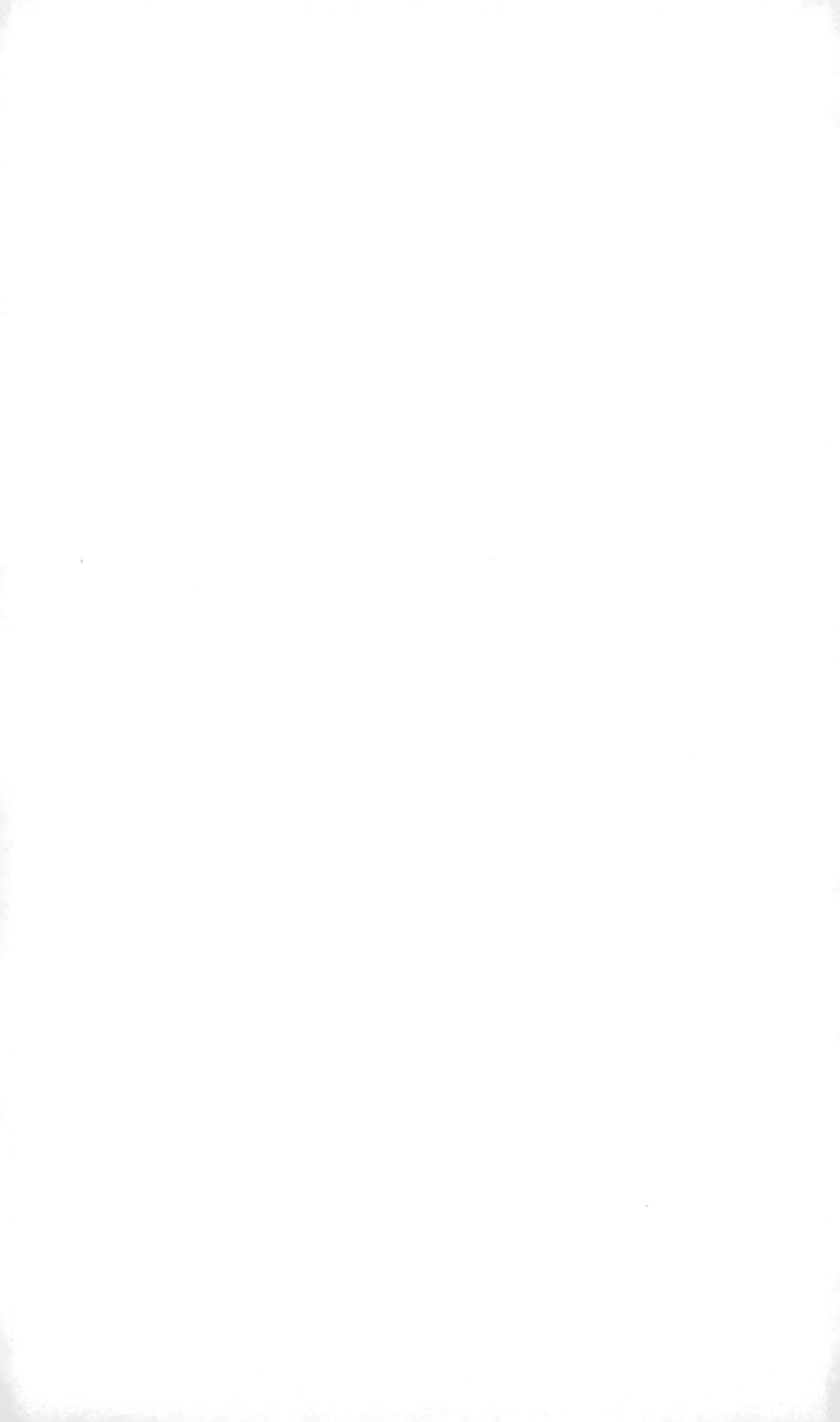

Church Attitudes on Sex from Antiquity

Without a doubt, the attitude of certain men in antiquity has affected the way we contemporary Christians look at sex. For many, sex was a nasty and dirty word that came only from Satan and not from God. Yet this way of thinking does not compute, because God, not Satan, is the one who initiated sex.

So since God kicked it off, why the distortion? In my own humble opinion, the distortion occurred because many church fathers were so (correctly) focused on spiritual things; they had a disregard (or little time) for fleshly things. In addition, yes, the flesh is bad, but not just in and of itself. When we eat, go to the bathroom, or follow other human urges, we act in the flesh. Make no doubt about that, but, in antiquity, this was not revealed. Many church fathers just wrote off sex and said it was only for procreation. In addition, that was it. Because of this, the caregivers of sex handed it over to Satan, and he has created what we have today.

Holy men, monks, and countless others practiced a piety that simply said, "No," to sex. Yes, sex is wrong outside of marriage, but in marriage, it is right. However, this was not the case with these holy men, and their beliefs influenced society to have sex only as it related to procreation. Anything outside of that was sinful, nasty, and most importantly, ungodly. Such views continue unto this day in some circles. Once again, we are told not to have sex outside of marriage, but within the frame of marriage, we can have it.

Along with demonizing, the libido came abuse of women. The train of thought goes something like this: because Eve disobeyed God first, she carries the weight of the original sin more than Adam does. Yet, I submit, it was Adam that the curse runs through, not Eve. If Adam had said, "No," the sin would not be here. The false prophets say that Eve incited Adam to eat the forbidden fruit; that is fine, but still, Adam had the power to make the right or wrong decision.

Men of antiquity became so overwrought about sex they took drastic actions. For instance, Origin of Alexandria (c. 185–c. 254) committed castration. Many have speculated that he did this so that he could tutor women in the area of sex. Yet, again, this was mainly because of his concern that he could not control the flesh. Had he just gotten married, this would not have been an issue at all.

According to Deschner's article, at some point the Catholic Church even tried to regulate the time and type of sex for married couples. This, in my opinion, is not godly or scripture based. She writes,

Even sex within the marriage was considered a sin, so the church started regulating it. In the early Middle ages this kind of filthy activity between married couples was forbidden on Sundays and other holydays, on days of penitence and prayer, on Wednesdays and Fridays, or Fridays and Saturdays, and of course in the forty-day long Fasting, in the four weeks of Advent, before going to Altar (*Eucharist*), under pregnancy, etc. (Deschner, 1987)[1]

Now, I do agree there are times that couples should give to the Lord, but the pastor or spiritual leader should not declare such times—especially when it comes to telling couples what they can and cannot do in the bedroom. The Bible again says that the marriage bed is honorable. If the bed is honorable for married people and bestowed by a loving God, why regulate or take it away?

The reason why I raise this is that there are people trying to regulate sex among couples today. This is truly ungodly and dangerous. If a man or woman can influence your sexual practices within the home, what is stopping them from taking it even further later on down the road?

In the same article, Deschner talks about the popes who said one thing but did other things. A prime example is Pope Alexander VI. This man had many mistresses while he was a priest. I bring up this point because many people who are all for piety are not practicing it themselves. Alternatively, they call others to a higher standard than they themselves do not follow.

When it comes to sex, some church leaders have tried to come off as holier as or mightier than others do, but when this happens, unsound teaching begins. Others popes did bad things, as did Pope Sixtus IV. He not only built the Sistine Chapel but also licensed a brothel. Here are a few other notes on issues relating to sex and the church:

An early law among Catholics said a married couple could be burned at the stake if they were caught having sex with the woman on top. Sex was only for conceiving children. For the male and, especially, the female to enjoy sex was not only deemed sinful, but could send them both to hell.

It will probably surprise you that Thomas Aquinas, another major influence in Christianity, felt that prostitution was unavoidable for a society.[2]

Given St. Augustine's strong anti-sex views, it will surprise and maybe baffle some that this sainted man felt that prostitution was necessary in society. He said, "If you expel prostitution from society you will unsettle everything on account of lusts."[3]

Augustine taught that procreation was the only non-sinful end of the sex act. He taught that if a couple has sexual relations for pleasure, they committed a venial sin. (According to Roman Catholicism, a venial sin, meaning a "forgivable" sin, is a lesser sin that does not result in a complete separation from God and eternal damnation in Hell. A venial sin involves a "partial loss of grace" from God.)

His precise words, from "On the Goods of Marriage" are:

Marital intercourse for the sake of procreation has no fault attached to it, but for the satisfying of lust, even with one's husband or wife, for the faith of the bed, is venially sinful; but adultery or fornication is mortally sinful. Moreover, continence from all intercourse is even better than marital intercourse itself, even if it takes place for the sake of procreation. However, even though continence is better, to pay the dues of marriage is no crime, but to demand it beyond the necessity of procreation is a venial sin, although fornication and adultery are mortally sinful.

Augustine commented on his sexual urges before he practiced celibacy, "What held me captive and tortured me was the habit of satisfying with vehement intensity an insatiable sexual desire" (*Confessions*, 6.12.22). For a bit more on Augustine's views on abstinence, here is part of *De Bono Conjugali*:

However, in good marriages among the elderly, although the glow of youth has withered between them, yet love between husband and wife still lives. <u>The better spouses they are, the earlier they have begun by mutual consent to abstain from sexual intercourse. Not that it should be necessary for them to do so, but it is praiseworthy for them to abstain</u>.

In other words, they do not have to have to abstain from intercourse, but it is good if they do so, and the earlier the better.

Our church fathers did their best when it came to sex, but I believe that each day we have a deeper revelation of things. I believe the time has come for married sexual couples to break the silence, be bold, and tell themselves that sex is good. The world has taken something that belongs to married couples, but the time has come to reverse this.

For more teaching by St. Thomas Aquinas on the subject of sex read Halsall, Paul. <u>Medieval Sourcebook</u>.1996. Fordham University. March 1996.<http://www.fordham.edu/halsall/source/aquinas-sex.html>

References
1. <http://www.bandoli.no/christianity_and_sex.htm\>
2. 1996–2007.<http://www.cybercollege.com/history.htm >
3. <http://www.bibletexts.com/qa/qa099.htm >

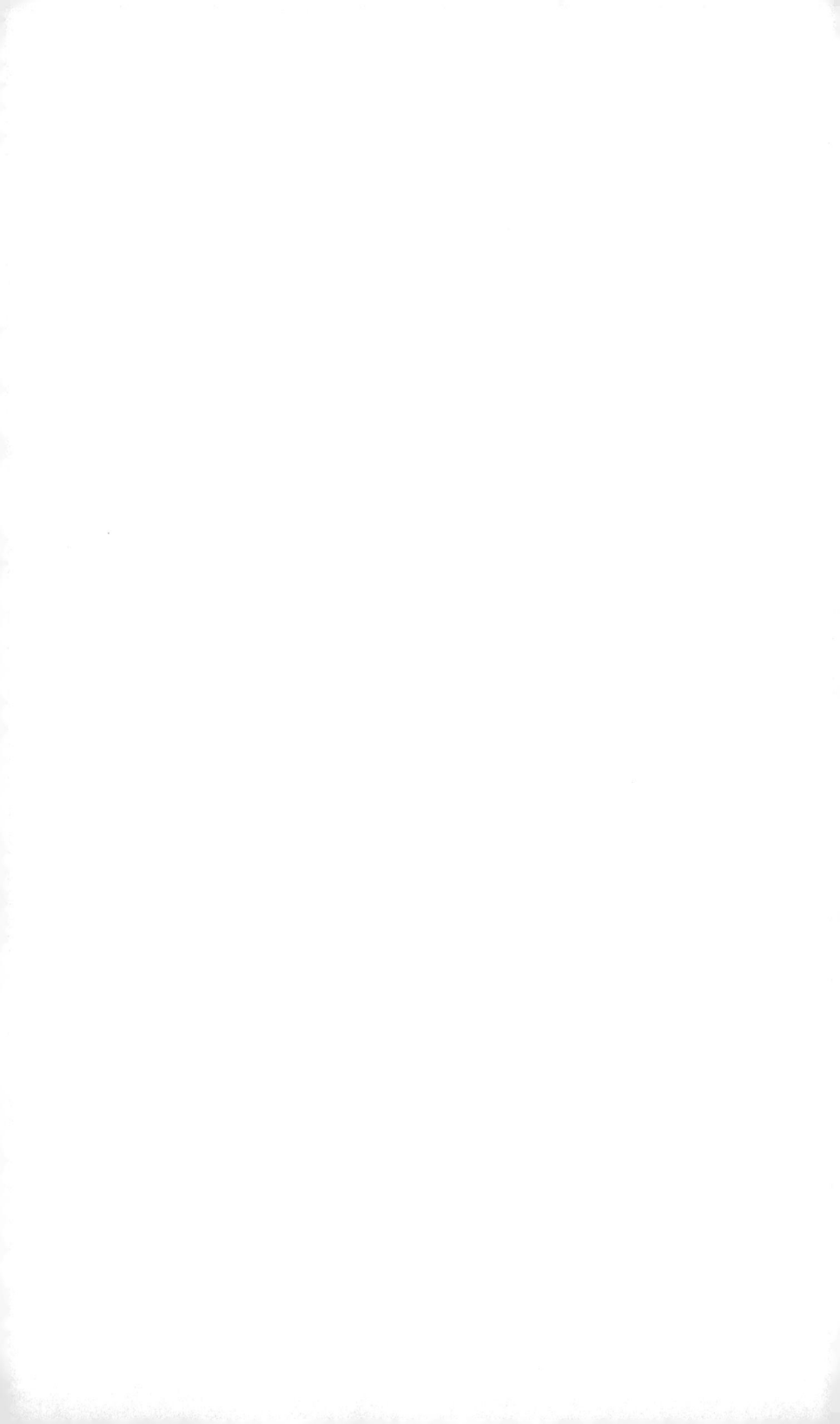

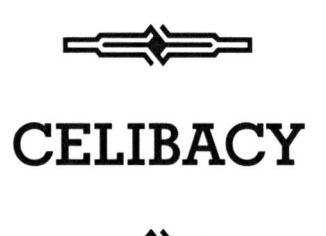

CELIBACY

Celibacy

By definition, *celibacy* is the absence of sexual intercourse for godly intentions. This is surely scripture based; however, once you are married, you must drop any idea of celibacy completely. The issue is that some discard the idea in the flesh, but not in the mind. Therefore, when the husband wants to get busy in the bedroom, he is treated as if he were a dog; or, if the wife desires sex, she is looked at as if she were a loose woman. Both perspectives need to be cleared up because celibacy and marriage are incompatible. They cover two different ends of the spectrum of sexuality.

Matthew 19 speaks of eunuchs, but eunuchs have no place in the marriage at all (or any place else, for that matter). Despite what other religious leaders have said, a sensual marriage is in God's eyesight beloved. If God preferred celibacy over marriage, he would have kept Adam single. However, HE saw that Adam was alone, and this alone time was not good for man in any shape or fashion. Because of this, when people put you down for being married and not celibate, you have a point of reference to direct the critic of married sex. Again, God created marriage and man created celibacy in a marriage environment. The devil is a liar.

In some churches, this is the rule of thumb. The second Lateran Council–Cannon 21(1139) made clerical marriages invalid[1]. Even Paul said that in the last days, people would condemn marriages; but this is not the will of God. The will of God is to believe in Him and Him alone and not make up things that are not there. Man is not the author; he is just the person who follows the rules of God. Yet men have tried repeatedly to make up things that are not there to prove their own righteousness. This has never been the will of God. The will of God is to follow His commandments and stay within the boundaries. When men try to add boundaries not given by God, they create false teachings and cults.

The celibacy question has always been debated in the Christian church because of the need to hate the flesh and love the spirit. This attitude to love the spirit and hate the flesh comes from the Greeks. Before the fall of man, there was man and woman. Before Genesis 3, there was Adam getting busy with Eve. Eve had sex with Adam.

In fact, the reason why God created Eve was for Adam to have sex with her. God said Adam's life was not good without woman. So why are we trying to change things for our own comfort and holiness level? Genesis 2:18 says, "I will make him a Help." The word *help* in Hebrew means 'aide.' Yes, we men need aid inside and outside of the bedroom.

We believe in celibacy for singles but not for married people. Celibacy and ascetic living is fine for the single person, but damnable for married couples.

Reference:
1. <http://www.answers.com/topic/first-council-of-the-lateran>

KNEW
(BIBLICAL WORD FOR SEX)

Knew (Biblical Word for Sex)

In the Old Testament, the word sex was never used. The word used for sex was knew, as in "Adam knew Eve." The word knew in Hebrew is yada. This means many things, including *observations, to know, to care, recognition, acknowledge, acquaintance, advise, certainty, discern, discover, feel, mark, perceive, have respect, and tell.*

Even in the Old Testament, God knew that just having sex was not enough. There were other things involved with and surrounding the physical act of a man and a woman coming together. I believe if each man and woman examines the original text of the word *knew*, marriages would be stronger. The problem is that our society only defines sex in the physical way.

The first translation of knew is *care*. When you have sex with your wife, you care. You are not just out for your own glory or what you desire but you are taking your love to another level because you say to yourself and your spouse, "It is not just about me, but about us." When there is no care or concern in the marriage, your marriage will fail. Again, we must look past the sex and see other issues that need to be addressed by the couple.

When you have sex without concern for your spouse, then the sex will be hindered, and you will not be able to take your love to the next level. In addition, after a while, the wife or husband will lose interest and, God forbid, find another. Therefore, there must be concern for each other. If you are hurting each other in or out of bed that is a legitimate concern that must be addressed. Such issues will cause problems down the road if they are ignored.

Another translation for knew in Hebrew (yada) is *recognition*. This is a bullet of a word because it goes to the significant part of understanding and recognizing what it is. Many couples fake or put up a smoke screen to avoid seeing the truth about their mate. They try not to accept the truth.

In most cases, an affair occurs when a couple does not really recognize the strength and weakness of the mate, and, of course, when they do not, they fall prey to the lust of others. Yet, when couples honestly face themselves and each other and say, "We will work this through," then you have the foundation for a great relationship and great sex.

In this section, I am really trying to convey that the sexual act is only the finished product. In other words, what I do outside the bedroom will affect goings on inside the bedroom. This is the reason for this book: the enormous fact that many Christians feel that as long as they love God and take care of the church, their spouses will love them dearly. Such is not the case. You must work on your marriage and not take it for granted.

The finished product (marriage) is not solely based

on sex. It is not solely based on the husband. It is not solely based on the wife. **It is based on love and forgiveness between married couples.** Therefore, if only one partner is working and the other partner is lazy, then you will have bad results. In addition, when I say couples should recognize each other for which they are, I do not mean the public image. I mean the people behind closed doors. Once this is done, they can see things in a clearer light.

The next translation for *knew* is *acknowledged*. To ignore one another is to keep each other in the dark from the love and sex needed in the marriage. Acknowledgement also goes to the point of acknowledging each other's needs and concerns. It is understanding each other's strengths and weaknesses.

It is not putting each other down and avoiding name-calling. It is lifting each other up. When couples lift each other, they both go higher. When you emotionally kill a spouse, you kill their self-esteem. When you acknowledge the other spouse, you learn something new about your spouse. This is a facet that many people do not comprehend: every time you are with your spouse, you are having a lesson. You are not just sitting there absorbing all the loving; you are learning and understanding the many needs of your spouse, which leads to a more perfect sex life.

The next word associated with sex (know) in the Hebrew is *acquaintance*. This is a very strong word because it means more than friendship. Couples have to be more than just friends with benefits are; they must be very well acquainted with each other. This only makes the bond of lovemaking stronger.

When husband and wife are just friends, they have

no strong bond between them; in reality, they are just roommates. Yet when they become acquaintances, they cannot only make physical love in the bedroom, but also they can make love with their thoughts and in the way, they treat one another. Many people mistake love for the flesh only, but true loving making is not just when you go to bed. It is on a day-in-and-day-out basis. In fact, the more foreplay you give your wife outside the bedroom, the easier it will be to have great sex in the bedroom.

Let me explain. Foreplay is not just touching in bed, but what you do outside the bedroom as well. If you touch your wife emotional and mentally, you will ensure something great. Like a running back, the more he touches, the better he runs. Well, husband, just as a note, your wife is a running back.

The more she is touched (sexually and non-sexually), the stronger she will become in her love for you. When you only give touches when you want to get some, you are making her cold and you are expecting her to warm up like a microwave; this is not the design of a woman. She needs touches. So, yes, brother, touch her morning, noon, and night. And, yes, wives, your husband does not mind being touched, either.

The word *advising* as a translation for *knowing* is a key one. When couples receive advice on their loving making, they are assured of many things. Most importantly, they are assured that the spouse will hear them when wisdom is given. They will not just have sex, but they will have each other's advice as they take their lives from one point to the next. In addition, advice is great in the bedroom.

Too many men are pig headed in not letting their wives take the lead in the bedroom. Does it not make sense to have the wife in charge of lovemaking since it takes her, on average, more time to reach orgasm? Does it not make sense to learn what makes her feel good?

Most husbands are just the opposite. Just one quick look can make husbands have orgasms. So, since men are fast and women are slow, it makes sense for her to advise her husband in the ways of loving making. <u>In essence, brothers when you are in bed and about to have sex, tell yourself, "Class is in session!"</u>

A marriage surely needs *certainty*. There needs to be strength in the marriage, and strength comes with the certainty spouses feel for one another. If one spouse thinks the other is cheating or not being forthright, then the lovemaking will be reserved and limited. Yet, if there is certainty in the marriage, now we have something going. When you know the brakes are off, you can ride freely without any hindrances at all. Many couples do not have great sex because they lack the feeling of certainty.

The husband is one day up and one day down. The wife is one day up and the next down. With this continued seesaw, nothing is final. Nothing is concrete. When you have a weak foundation, you cannot expect to grow. You cannot expect to do great things. With certainty, you will have a foundation that ensures loving in all types of matters and conditions. This is what is needed in the marriage: certainty that you will keep your vows and love no matter what. Husband, one thing that wives need on an ongoing basis is a lot of certainty; they need to know that you are theirs totally and completely. Once this is established, the loving making will be established as well.

The word *discern* has gotten a bad rap. Many feel this word is for the super-spiritual or the especially discerning, but in actuality, it is associated with every couple. This is especially true for the wives. Husbands will agree with me that when you try to hide something from your wife, this is when it will become fully discovered. Most wives have the discerning gene. This is why men you cannot just have sex with her and continue to deny her discerning abilities. When you say, "No," when the answer is "Yes," you do nothing but cause problems in your bedroom.

I have heard this over time: "My husband does not listen to me. I warn him and he goes on down the road anyway." The wife may say, "Pastor, it seems he does not respect my skills to discern." However, a smart husband will respect this in his wife. A smart husband will learn to take his wife's super powers and use them to help the family go to the next level.

Even more importantly, when the wife knows that the husband has confidence in her abilities, she is much more likely to let him use his sexual powers on her. Too many husbands have missed the opportunity for great loving because they did not listen to their wives and respect their God-given abilities. This must change for bedroom activity to rise to another level.

The word *discover* is a beautiful word. Yet, this word does not just relate to the bedroom, it relates to all facets of the marriage. Many times men fail to see the power of discovering their wife. When you fail to discover all the things about her that is when you will fall prey to affairs or a lack of love and respect toward your wife. This is unhealthy. Everyday is an adventure with your wife.

Everyday she does something different that just rocks our world. Everyday she speaks words that we have never heard before. Just as you want to discover new ways of making love and new avenues of sex within your marriage, you first must have own your Indiana Jones's hat and whip. Just as Dr. Jones found new adventures, we can find new adventures with our wives.

Yes, I did say 'whip' a minute ago, but the whip is not for you, it is really for her as she tames you to learn her desires and teaches you to pleasure her. In fact, couples can share the whip as they discover one another. She uses it outside the bedroom and you use it inside the bedroom, brothers. This is how it moves accordingly and in motion. Wives, this is your opportunity to show love and teach him how to love and discover you. Meanwhile, husbands, in the bedroom you use the whip to show your wife another side of loving making. Again, remember, the whip is a symbol you get to use together as you discover and share one another.

The next word is *feeling*. This word is surely foreign to most men. A wife must feel your love and not just your touch. Many husbands know how to feel up their wives, but that is not the same as the wife feeling your love for her. If her mind is one way and you are other way, she is not going to reach an orgasm.

Her mind must be in tune with yours. If her mind is on other things, she is not gong to be comfortable. This is another reason why so many wives take a long time to heat up. They take long because they must divert their minds from what they were thinking before you pushed up against them and suggested having sex. Women are multi-taskers. Yet, many times the last thing on their mind is sex. Once you learn these men, you will become better in the bedroom.

For God's sake, do not ask her what she is feeling. Instead, if you get to know your wife, she will not have to say how she is feeling. You will know it by yourself. Men, this is key. The key is to feel up your wife. No, I am not taking about her breasts and thighs; I am talking a little higher. I am talking about her (brain) feelings.

She also could be feeling that she does not love her body any more, and she is trying to wrap her brain around the idea that 10 years ago, she was a size 4, and now, after the babies, she is a size 10+. In fact, before you hit the sack to have sex, find out how she is feeling. Remember men; operate the mind, then her body.

The next word for *know* or *sex* in the bible that we will examine is *mark*. To some this may seem weird but in actuality, it is not. Here we are talking about knowing that both husband and wife are marked only for each other and nobody else. So many times wives cannot make that love making transaction because she questions if you are marked for her, meaning no other woman can touch you but her.

This is nothing but good old-fashioned ownership. Some men wonder if they are the only one for her. This is why you mark each other: you say, "No one can cross this border but me. No one can touch, taste, or handle that sexual organ—only I can do that." Once that mark is made and secure in the minds of wife and husband, the lovemaking will not only continue but also it will blossom. As long as there is ambiguity in the relationship, the lovemaking cannot and will not flourish.

The next word relating to sex is *perceived*. The word means to really know what is going on and not have secrets between each other. All persons have a private versus public personality, but spouses cannot have this in marriage. They must be very transparent to one another. They cannot hide from each other.

The next word we will examine is *respect*. This is a very strong word. If a wife feels she has no respect from her husband, she cannot free herself sexually. She will always hold back. She will never let go for her husband because she will wonder, as the old movies asked, "Will you respect me in the morning." This is a powerful question in many ways. When you have stripped a wife of her respect, what does she have?

We all remember the force field that Star Trek fighters used to defend themselves from invaders. Respect is the force field for woman, and when that force field is down, and then all types of things are exposed. Husbands, when the wife says, "No sex tonight," the answer is "No." You may beg, borrow, or steal, but you must respect your wife's wishes. The wife must also respect her husband's wishes. Yes, marriage is surely a give-and-take proposition. If you do not love and respect, you will not get it in return.

The last word we will cover is *told*. Without a doubt, this is the most powerful because the word relates to communicating. If couples only communicate when it is time for sex or time to argue, there will be no good sex. In my books, I express to men the power of telling versus the power of being told.

There is nothing more powerful than a wife hearing from her husband his desires as there is nothing like a husband's hearing his wife's desires. When both of these things are met, you have power and love to the fullest. When you do this and talk to each other, the bedroom activities will flow much easier.

When you apply the above words, sex will move from causal to the unbelievable.

SEX ON THE BRAIN: RELEASING HORMONES

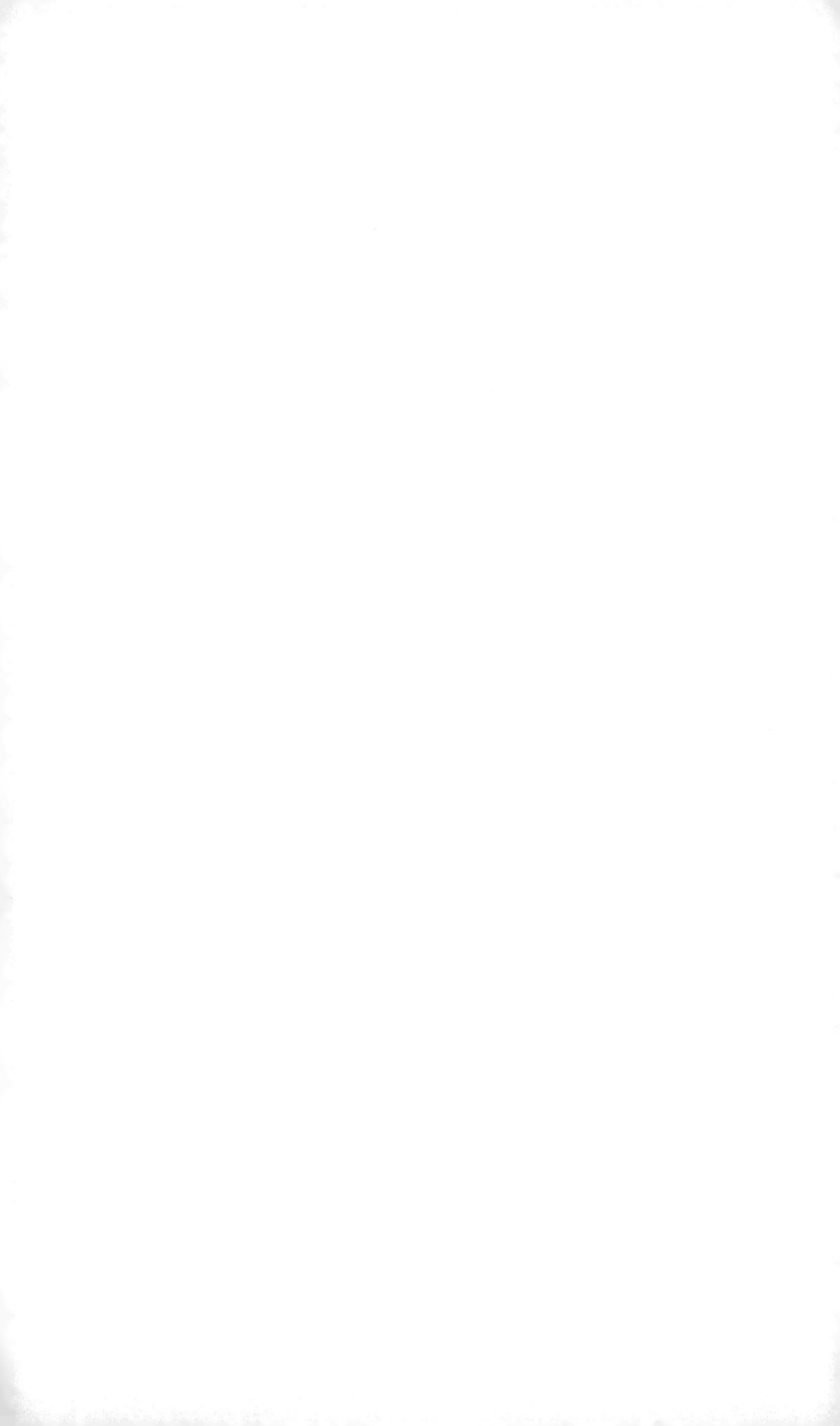

SEX on the Brain: Releasing Hormones

In my quest to help married couples understand that sex came from God himself, I must take a detour and look at the human body and, in particular, the brain. The brain is the same for both Christians and sinners. The only thing that changes upon conversion is the way one thinks and processes information. A sinner will process for himself while a Christians (should) process for the glory and honor of God. This is the big difference between the two.

Guilt may be the only major difference in emotions that people have during sex; one having sex in marriage feels no guilt while one having sex outside marriage will feel guilt. In sum, a Christian who commits adultery or fornication will have guilt accompanying loving making because that Christian is breaking the laws of God.

Those committing fornication, adultery, homosexuality, or heterosexually married sex will all experience a release of hormones and brain activities during the act of sex. I mention this because once you understand that God created sex and gave us these feelings, it is less of an argument to convince married Christians that sex is all right. Some have feelings during the act and automatically think they have sinned, but in this section, I will show you that the feelings and hormone release are not the sin, it is the vehicle that releases them (fornication vs. heterosexual married sex).

Let us take the ungodly, unholy, and criminal act of a woman being raped. Some women who have been sexually assaulted feel guilt after such an assault because during the criminal assault they felt pleasure. Grantley Morris writes, "When one's body involuntarily sends pleasure signals to the brain in response to sexual molestation, it says nothing about one's morality or attitude towards the offense."[1]

Some people even reach orgasm while being violated. This is because the brain automatically starts functioning in a sexual mode once the engine starts to turn. From these ungodly situations, some women who have been molested or raped carry guilt in their souls. For those who are married, the husband may be unaware of why his wife does not want to get sexual with him. It is not because she hates him; it is possible she does not want to associate the orgasm of her godly union with her husband with the orgasm she had during the rape.

This is like walking in a minefield, to say the least; especially if one's first sexual experience was one of molestation, rape, or sexual abuse. The wife and husband will first have to come to terms with this issue, and then take it to counseling to help dissect the feelings involved.

Grantley Morris continues:

Victims of sexual crime often suffer horrific, but unnecessary pangs of guilt over being forced to experience pleasure. Having a nice feeling in the midst of rape or molestation is usually no more than a bodily reaction like bleeding. It in no way suggests the person is immoral or subconsciously wants to be abused. And any skilled seducer of children will have much about him or her that normal children are drawn too.

This is unnecessary guilt and it is sweeping our country. Women who have been abused take such memories into a marriage with them, and then both husband and wife suffer. The release of sexual hormones is not the sin; it is the method that creates the release. I know I have given an extreme example in rape, but the point is that during the act of sex, the body, which God made, will release hormones to experience the pleasure points.

Yes, some Christians feel that feeling pleasure while in the act of sex is wrong; it is not wrong. It is good. Since God made everything we have, including our body parts, then it is time for us to stop denying what God has given to every healthy, normal human being. In the following excerpts, other experts weigh in on the subject of rape and sexual assault:

A woman's physiological responses to sexual contact are involuntary and in no way imply consent. A woman can become aroused, lubricate, and even orgasm against her will during a rape. Furthermore, even if orgasm during rape is intensely physically pleasurable for the victim, it can lead to great stress afterwards if the victim comes to associate physical pleasure with the trauma of rape.[2]

In fact, when sexual stimulation starts, the feelings and the release of hormones are totally out of the person's control. This is why I try to make this point that both sinner and saint will have a release of emotions, but, remember, it is how the release is done. Now that I have made that point, let's go into the functions of the brain while having sex.

Oxytocin is a hormone within every human, and it is known to help form relationships. This hormone comes into play during childbirth, breast feeding, and sex. Oxytocin is a relatively small peptide hormone composed of only nine amino acids and is secreted from the posterior lobe of the pituitary gland.[3] Its major function is to help the mother during labor, and its second function is producing milk for the baby. These two actions reflect the close relationship a wife has with her husband. One, she is producing a baby with his sperm. She shows her commitment to the man by going through childbirth, and then after the baby is born, she feeds the child from her breasts.

Yet, in its true sense, Oxytocin is released during coitus or intercourse. As most people know, when the penis is within the vagina, the uterus contracts, which again releases the hormone. This is the same for sinner and saint—it happens in all healthy females. (Males also release Oxytocin, but its role in men is not clear. Some say that Oxytocin facilitates male sperm as they race toward the uterus.) The point is the hormones are released during sex and child bearing.

The word *Oxytocin* in Greek means *quick birth*. Furthermore, in humans, Oxytocin is released during orgasm in both sexes. In the brain, Oxytocin is involved in social recognition and bonding, and might be involved in the formation of trust between people. Oxytocin increases trust in humans.[4]

For most humans, the level of Oxytocin is especially high in the morning, which is why, according to Ilia Karatsoreos, Ph.D.[5], levels of Oxytocin (known as the love hormone) are sky high upon waking up. Hence, this makes it the best time for intimacy. There is no denying it; this is the way God planned it. Romans chapter 1 tells us nature shows the power and wealth of God. Since childbirth is natural and comes from God, how can I possibly say pleasure between husband and wife is wrong? No, sir, I cannot, and neither can anyone else. Remember, in Genesis 18:12, even Sarah desired pleasure. The word *pleasure* in the Hebrew is *Eden* or *ednah*. This is translated as *delight* or *pleasure*. God is not the one who waves a club and condemns husband and wife when they pleasure each other sexually. No, this has been the doing of man because he did not understand the nature of God.

Couples, do you have any idea how many sensory nerve endings are within the clitoris compared to the penis? Over one hundred times more! Married couples can find ways to satisfy themselves and release more Oxytocin between them on a day-in-and-day-out basis to create and enhance the bonding between man and wife.

Endorphins, natural aspirins for the body, are released into the blood stream to help relieve pain. Researchers tell us that strenuous exercise stimulates this process.[6] Even better for us, others have found that we release endorphins during orgasm, as well as during laughter. In fact, a large dose of endorphins is released during lovemaking. This release is not based on the state of one's soul—saved or unsaved—it is a biological blessing that God gave man and woman. The point I want to make is that God gave us a way to have a release in our lives and many Christians do not use it. Instead of going to the medicine chest, it may be time to go to the bedroom. It is time to look at the natural way of relieving pain called sex.

If God gave sex to Adam and Eve, why does the Christian world rebuke married couples for enjoying a God-given gift? This is the very definition of being sexually repressed. Husband and wife, your Heavenly father gave you sex, not just to create babies, but also to relieve the stress that we face in our lives. Endorphins also reduce stress and affect our emotions.[7] In fact, the word *endorphin* stands for endomorphine. This is the human drug that God gave husbands and wives to endure pain within their lives. It is not a sin to release endorphins during sex; it is only a sin if you are not with your husband or wife.

Another source asks,

Why would a natural analgesic occur during something as pleasurable as sex? Endorphins (and elevated serotonin levels) cause "runner's high", a release, which occurs due to necessary pain alleviation in stressed muscles. Invigorating sex is exertion, and therefore causes the same release. Intense pleasure also relates to pain; women often have the same extroverted and chemical, reactions in child birth as they do during sex. You know those moments when you feel like it is just too much, but you are loving it and don't ever want to stop? Some people release endorphins during orgasm, others do so from non-climactic over-stimulation.[8]

The point I want to secure in your mind is that God has given us something to help deal with our lives. We do not need drugs or alcohol, married couples. The only thing you need is to get into bed and get busy.

Even *Forbes* magazine understands the importance of sex. The magazine reports one of the many good qualities of sex is

Pain-relief: Immediately before orgasm, levels of the hormone Oxytocin surge to five times their normal level. This in turn releases endorphins, which alleviate the pain of everything from headache to arthritis to even migraine. In women, sex also prompts production of estrogen, which can reduce the pain of PMS.[9]

In fact, the greater the activity, the higher the level of

endorphins entering the blood stream. When people go into shock, endorphins work within the body to help regulate it until medical support comes. Well, if God planned it that way, why are we waiting to enjoy something that God has given? Pleasure, my married Christian couples, is not wrong. God intended us to have a pleasure valve, and he gave it to all of us. Couples please stop denying or refuting something, God has given. To rebuke pleasure between married couples is to rebuke God. Why? God made the pleasure, so why deny the pleasure of the pain reliever.

DHEA (dehydroepiandrostone) is a hormone that keeps one young. Even better, it enters the blood stream during sex. Let us look at this, married couples, as God has given us, free of charge, the fountain of youth. There is no other way to look at it. The Lord has given us back the Garden of Eden by giving us the DHEA hormone when we have great sex with hour spouses.

A 1994 study by researchers at the University of California, San Diego, looked at 30 middle-age men and women who took 50 mg of DHEA a day for three months. The test subjects generally reported an improved sense of well-being, increased energy, enhanced libido, and an improved ability to deal with stress. The results were widely reported by the mass media, with several referring to DHEA as the "fountain of youth hormone."[10]

Forget the plastic surgery and botox, and hear the Lord when He says: find a mate of the opposite sex, marry and commit, and have great sex. Not only will it bless you and pleasure you, it will also keep you young.

The problem is, because we Christians have hidden under the sheets when it comes to sex, we have given the world permission to take over what God commanded married heterosexuals to do. However, not only did we hide, but also the world has prospered from something that God gave married couples. We must reclaim our rights to this area. We cannot continue to be idle on this matter.

According to William Regelson, M.D., a specialist in medical oncology at the Medical College of Virginia, he says "by restoring one's DHEA levels to their youthful equivalent, an aging person can improve their memory, rejuvenate their immune system, increase their overall physical energy, reduce body fat, prevent heart disease, and enhance their libido".[11]

In other words, if you return your DHEA levels to your 25-year-old levels, you might feel as if you have reversed the aging process. God made DHEA levels high during our youth because it is the best time, physically, for procreating and child rearing. Yet, after a certain age, that same DHEA can keep a body young. It may not produce a baby, but it will produce pleasure in one who is older, and that is a good thing. More information on DHEA follows:

DHEA is converted into testosterone, which is known to enhance libido in both men and women. This helps to explain why so many people report heightened sexual desire after they begin taking DHEA supplements. However, there may be more to DHEA's enhancement of sexual desire and performance than simply raising testosterone levels. Because taking DHEA raises the levels of all adrenal hormones, it tends to make people feel more energetic, and enhances feelings of well-being in general. It also tends to improve overall heath, and anything that improves physical health and well-being is likely to reflect positively on one's sexual health as well.[12]

The information below[13], illustrates some actions, reactions, and functions of the brain during sex:

viewing erotic images affects the **interior and middle frontal gyri**

insula is activated during erections

brain activity, such as that in the **median preoptic** area, is essential to sexual performance

medical amygdala and hypothalamus regulate sexual behavior boosting primal urges

God has provided all of these brain activities, and, as I said earlier, it affects sinner and saint alike. The key, however, is to ensure what type of stimuli is setting the brain into action. Some may disagree, but I think it is all right for a man to have erotic images of his wife. Men, be honest. We all have images in our head—the key is to take the body and make it your wife's. Doing so will ensure your are not lusting after the wrong flesh.

The following includes more information about your brain during sex:

> Although you think everything happens between your legs, the sensation of orgasm actually originates between your ears, in the form of chemical messengers and the receptors they bind to. These neurochemical changes take place in the limbic system, or "mammalian brain." The mammalian brain controls almost all bodily functions. It's the seat of emotions, desires, drives and impulses.
>
> The more dopamine you release and the more your reward center is activated, the more "reward" you experience. You're craving the dopamine that is

released with these activities. Dopamine is your major motivation, not the item or activity.

Researchers placed electrodes in rats' reward centers to stimulate them, just as dopamine does. The rats could then press a lever to stimulate the reward center. That's all those rats did; they ignored food, and even female rats. They just sat there pressing the lever over and over, wasting away...not unlike crack addicts. In a second experiment, scientists blocked dopamine so the reward center could not be stimulated. What happened? The rats just sat there, again ignoring food, receptive mates, and the opportunity to explore their environment. Orgasm is the biggest blast of dopamine (legally) available to us. A Dutch scientist recently scanned the brains of people having orgasm. He said they resembled scans of heroin rushes. He saw visions of an "orgasm pill" and lots of money. We saw visions of one of the most <u>addictive substance ever produced</u>.

Orgasms and addictions have two things in common. They both produce an initial pleasurable experience, and both are followed by an unpleasant hangover. The sexual satiation (orgasm) hangover is innate. It can be such a subtle part of you that you do not connect the dots--unless you switch to making love without it for several weeks, and then go back to sex with orgasm. "What goes up must come down." It's simple biology; body systems must return to balance, or homeostasis. What goes up and down in this case is your dopamine. That can play havoc with your <u>mood</u> and the way in which you perceive, and treat, your partner.[14]

I hope I leave you with the message that we cannot

accept only certain parts of God. Yes, God is wrathful, but He is also the Creator of dopamine, sex and pleasure. We cannot take certain things God offers us and discard others. That's what Humanists do; they love creation but hate the Creator. They want all the rights and riches of humanity, but they give no honor to the Creator.

Just as a prophet has no honor in his country, so God has no honor in His creation. Either He is getting dismissed by atheists or He is limited by zealous Christians who think of God as holy but ignore or diminish what He bestowed on married heterosexual creatures. You cannot have it both ways. I know God created us. How can I turn around and say, "Oh yeah, you did good, God, but the sensual pleasure between husband and wife is not Godly." If the brain is created by God, and it works the same way with everyone, then we cannot deny the workings of the Lord. We cannot say "He did not create sex." No, Christians, God made sex for married couples, and we should enjoy it to the fullest.

Reference
1. Morris, Grantley. <http://net-burst.net/hope/abuse_pleasure.htm>
2. Amen, Daniel. Sex on the Brain: 12 Lessons to Enhance Your Love Life. Three Rivers Press. 2008
3. <(http://www.answers.com/topic/oxytocin?cat=health>
4. Nature International Weekly Journel of Science. Oxytocin increases trust in humans 2005.<http://www.nature.com/nature/journal/v435/n7042/abs/nature03701.html>
5. Prevention Magazine (June 2008), and Karatsoreos, Ilia. Let Your Brain Reign. April 2008. Prevention

Magazine. <http://www.prevention.com/cda/article/let-your-brain-reign/afd043310886911OVgnVCM10000013281eac___/?print=true>
6. <http://www.goaskalice.columbia.edu/0483.html>
7. <http://www.answers.com/topic/endorphin->
8. Sailing, Jasmine. Endorphins: Free Smack!. #2 of *Morbid Curiosity*, Automatism Press < http://cyberpsychos.netonecom.net/jsailing/actual/heroin.html >
9. Gisquet, Vanessa. Better Sex Diet. 2005.Forbes Magazine.<http://www.forbes.com/2005/03/17/cx_vg_0317feat.html>
10. < http://www.answers.com/topic/dhea>
11. Brown, David J Sex and DHEA <http://www.sexanddrugs.info/dhea.htm.>
12. DHEA Supplements: What Are They and Are They Safe?<http://www.webmd.com/a-to-z-guides/dhea-supplements>
13. *Men's Health Magazine* (July/August 2008)
14. <http://www.reuniting.info/science/sex_in_the_brain>

LINGERIE AND SEXY UNDERWEAR

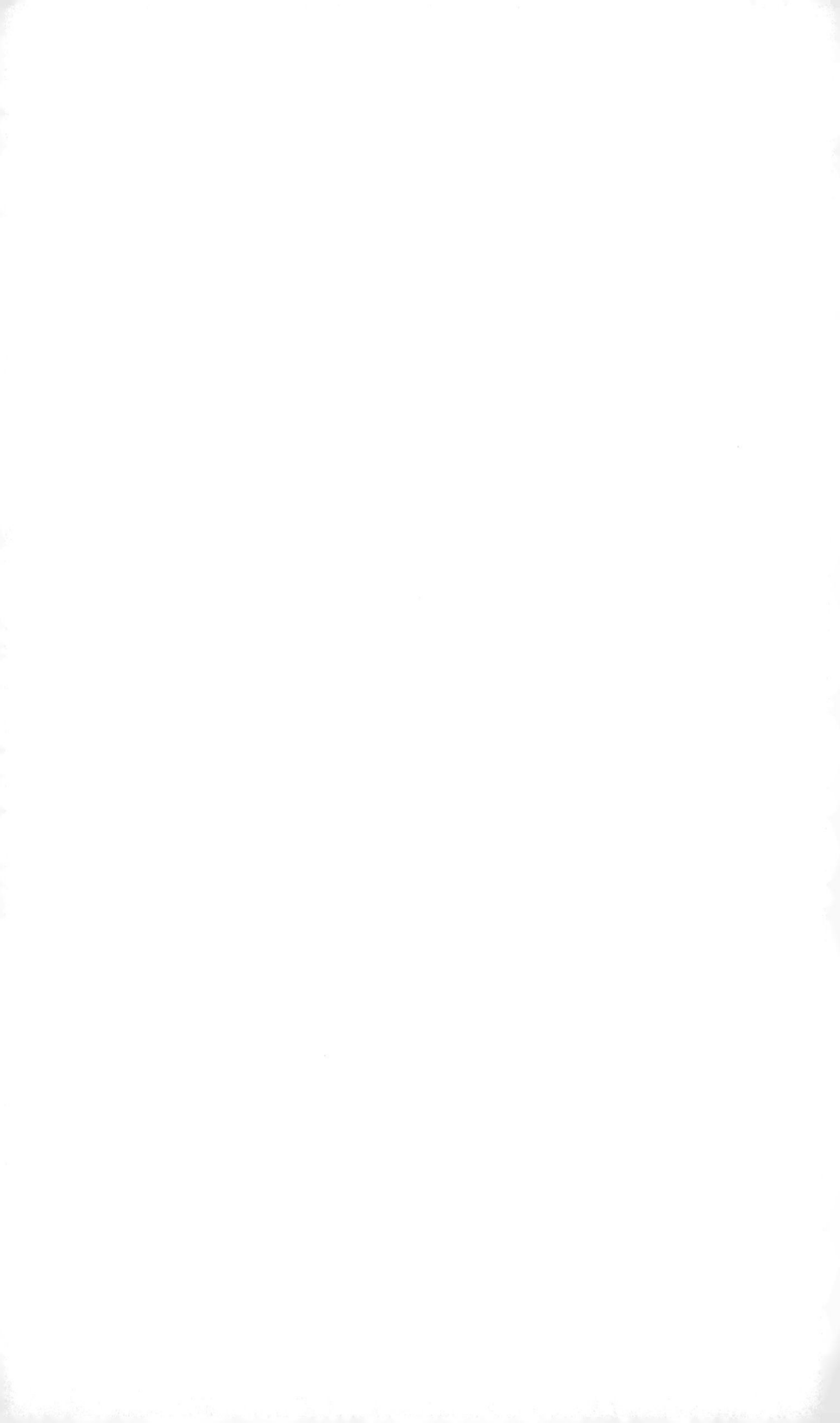

Lingerie and Sexy Underwear

Some in the church feel that wearing sexy lingerie is ungodly and goes against the plan of God. Some feel that because worldly people wear sexy lingerie, it is wrong to do so. Nevertheless, if you follow my logic, if it is cool to dress well in the business world, how much cooler is it to do so in the bedroom?

Shouldn't we want to impress our mates? Shouldn't we want to look good for them? Too often, I hear Christians who dress well for the world, but for their husbands or wives, they dress like bums. I rebuke this and protest against it. If you are going to put your best foot forward for the world, then you should do the same for your spouse. Yes, this means lingerie and sexy underwear.

Women, dressing in a sexy way does not make you a slut (you make the clothes; the clothes do not make you). You are not slutty for dressing in sexy items for your man, wives. Now I agree, some things should be done or worn only inside the home and not in sight of the whole world, but do not let that be an excuse for not wearing certain things for your mate.

Have you heard people say you dress the way you want to feel? I agree. If you want to feel sexy and be attractive to your mate, then dress accordingly. Some couples do not even try to spice up their relationship. This is not fair or correct. This must be turned around. When you give each other your bodies in the bedroom, present yourself in the best possible light.

In fact, if couples presented themselves this way, they might fight less and make love more often. For example, men, if you look messy from the feet up, you have to expect your wife to act accordingly. However, if you come dressed as if you love and desire your spouse, she may love and desire you in return.

Wives, men are visual creatures. This is why the average man watches porn—he likes to see. If you want him to see you more, then you have to dress accordingly. It amazes me how we, as Christians, can be blind to some worldly things, but other worldly things we adapt to eagerly. For example, a computer is worldly. It is what you do with it that can take if from good to evil. However, nearly all of us have one in our homes or we use one on the job. Well, the same concept applies in wearing sexy clothing for each other.

The porn industry is a $3 billion industry, and men are drawn to it like moths to a flame. Yet, Christian women do not take the hint. I am not saying you should watch porn to become a star, but you understand the importance of romance and wearing sexy things. It is not a sin. You are only making yourself appetizing to your mate. There is no sin in that.

You can use different sexy clothing to spice up the day and not the same old thing that hides everything that God has given you. In addition, speaking of hiding things, ladies, and a husband who is into you will love every part of you including the baby marks on your body. Many women try to hide their bodies. Be open, completely open, about the things in and through your life. Dress for love and not for hate.

Dress for your mate. Wear the clothing as if it is coming off any way, and it will. I know you do not want your wife or husband to fantasize alone. So, if you do not want that to happen, why not give him or her dream to live. Why not say, "Honey, I am yours. I am what you want me to be. How do you want me to be today in the bedroom?" Do not hold back, but let yourself fall totally into the love that God has given you.

Before we end this chapter, I want to tell wives once more: you must become comfortable in your body. In this book, we spoke about the fears of many, but the fear that stops many women is the way they view their own bodies. Women, if you are not comfortable with your own body in front of your husband that will inhibit great sex.

While your husband is trying to love on you, you are wondering what he is thinking of this mark or that blemish on your body. Wives, I will speak from love that is the last thing on the mind of a man who really loves you. He is not worried about the marks and other little flaws you see. He just wants you and you alone.

This gives women another reason to wear sexy clothing for their husband; it helps them dress things up and makes them feel sexier about their own bodies. When you put on certain clothing or certain accessories, you feel differently and stop stressing about the way you look. Your husband wants you, and when he married you, he married all of you. So, stop stressing.

You will communicate your stress to your mate. If you feel unsexy, he is going to take his attention elsewhere, which is not what you want. So, wear clothes that make you feel better. The sexy clothing industry can help make any women at any size look great. Yes, I said it. You may have to go to some specialty shop, but wives, the clothing is out there for you to look good in.

Husbands, if you desire your wives to wear sexy clothing, you must encourage them. In fact, a smart man will find out what his wife thinks about her body and why. Why does she feel inhibited by her body? What is making her not want to be sexual? This is the time for love and patience and not ruling with an iron fist. This is the time for the love and passion that must take place in and throughout your life. When you take that time for each other, then you will make each other better.

ARGENTINE LAKE DUCK
(SIZE CAN SCARE YOU)

Argentine Lake Duck (Size Can Scare You)

This chapter is very important because too many men—whether saved or not—have issues with penis size. In fact, some wives worry about their husband's penis size as well. The pornography industry has made the size of a man's penis a hot topic, and when a man measures five inches (average), he thinks he does not have what it takes to please his wife, but he does.

God gave every husband enough to satisfy the longing of his wife. This is a moot point: it is not the size, but the action of the penis in the vagina. To get my point across, I will talk about the animal kingdom as it relates to large sex organs. Most of my information on this comes from an article by Hilary Mayell of *National Geographic News*.[1]

Zoologists believe that the Argentine Lake Duck has the largest sex organ (17 inches) on a mammal. Unbelievably, the duck weighs only 640 grams and extends 16 inches. In other words, the duck's penis is as long as the duck itself. I cannot imagine any wife wanting her husband to have a penis as long as he is tall. Such a nightmare would drive any wife out of the bedroom. If this is true, why do we overemphasize penis size? It is because we have lost focus.

Mayell's article continues, the base of the Argentine Lake Duck's penis is covered with coarse spines, while the tip is soft and brush-like. The researchers think a drake may use the brush-like tip as a sort of cleansing instrument before ejaculation to remove sperm in the female's oviduct that was deposited by another suitor, thus increasing the mating drake's chances of paternity.

In essence, every male may be trying to do that same thing: remove the memories of other men from his wife's past before he met her. Men are very competitive and always trying to one up each other. However, I tell men, there is no competition.

The other men did not have the commitment or the balls to stay after they made love. Yes, commitment is stronger than lovemaking. Therefore, instead of erasing your wife's memory of old suitors, make history together so that she no longer remembers her old suitors by your commitment to her.

Because the Argentine Duck's penis is so long, this bird is ALWAYS promiscuous; it is not a monogamous creature. So let us take this further. To the wife who desires her husband's penis to be longer, there is a possibility that that husband with a huge penis might stray and become promiscuous.

Likewise, to the husband who wants a bigger penis, you may be tempted to stray from your wife and become promiscuous. In addition, a large member at times makes men overly confident in the bedroom, and this is a difficult issue to overcome. I want you to understand the importance of accepting what you have and the package God has given you.

Dr. McCracken also mentions that the Duck's penis might be used as a lasso to catch females. Now this is deep. The duck uses his penis to bring a female closer. In reality, human men do the same. When you make great love with your wife, you help her release hormones that will draw her, or lasso her, emotionally closer to you. In no way is this done physically, but, more importantly, it must be done mentally, emotionally, and psychologically. Many husbands do not realize that a wife's most sensitive love organ is her brain. Once you love her emotionally, you have her physically.

Reference
1. National Geographic News. May 18, 2009 < http://news.nationalgeographic.com/news/2001/10/1023_corkscrewduck_2.html >

WARNING: YOUR MEMBER HAS AN EXPIRATION DATE; RENEW IT!

WARNING: Your Member Has an Expiration Date; Renew It!

Our lives have an expiration date. Every person who is born has a time designed by God to check out of this life. Life is what you do between checking in and checking out. Since this is the case, married couples must learn to renew their sexual and communication skills constantly.

When couples get in a certain mind frame as it relates to sex and communication, the expiration date is coming. Smart couples will constantly keep the expiration date at bay, they will renew their relationship. Let us look at milk. A carton of milk includes an expiration date. You cannot change that date stamped on the carton. You can decide to ignore it, but the milk will spoil. The consumer has two decisions: 1) drink the milk before the expiration date or 2) pour out the milk after the date.

Couples, it is the same thing with your marriage. When it comes to sex and communication, there is an expiration date—the time when the way you do things gets boring and monotonous. Smart couples will notice when things are getting old and take the necessary steps to step up

| 247

the game. When I say expiration, I mean when things are old and nothing seems new. You cannot let your communication or sex become spoiled; each couple must find ways to keep it fresh.

I do not believe in divorce, except for extreme cases including affairs; for this reason, couples must keep the vagina and penis fresh so their relationship does not spoil. They must keep their communication fresh to avoid the pitfalls of life. How do you keep things fresh? You have a constant renewing of the mind. You constantly talk about the last time you loved or communicated and from that conversation, you make important adjustments.

No couple is perfect. No couple will have all the points in play all the time. You must find ways to keep the marriage in order. This may mean dressing differently or talking of different things to keep you both fresh and interesting. Whether hair, nails, dress or whatever it takes, a wife can make sure her husband will see a new woman everyday. When you keep the target moving, you keep the marriage moving as well. In addition, yes, the husband must move the target as well for his wife interest.

No woman wants to wear the same old outfit forever, and men eventually want a new car because he's had the old car long enough, and it's time for an upgrade. Since I do not believe in upgrade in the sense of divorce, I suggest a renewing of the mind. It is a renewing of the way things are done to keep things fresh.

Smart couples must keep communication and sex alive and fresh. Without freshness of communication and sex, the marriage will get old. Then it is ready for retirement. You may laugh at what I am saying, but you must keep things interesting and renewed. If you do not, then retirement will happen. When retirement comes as it relates to communication and sex, then divorce or affairs are soon to follow.

A way to keep the marriage fresh is to first know what you like and do not like. It is time to stop hiding behind shame and religion, know you, and then know each other. Couples must fight the natural urge to just let things be. Only God is being; couples are becoming. In other words, couples should change and get better and better everyday. Do not sit still and wait for death or divorce, but find ways to keep things fresh.

In fact, couples, try to keep physical and emotional orgasms going. Some couples find ways to sustain the love and feelings that they have for each other. If you do nothing, you will get nothing; however, if you do something, you will get great results. If you do nothing and expect something, you are foolish. Life is nothing but cause and effect. There can be no effect unless there is a cause. When you have a cause, then you get an effect.

Couples must make things happen or things will happen on their own. As they gracefully age, they must have ways to keep the emotional and sexual going strong. I have spoken about this in other books, but if we use physical aids, then so be it: it is time to use sexual aids that you have agreed upon.

When our eyes get dim or the body needs additional hormones, we have no problem in using eyeglasses, canes, or supplements to maintain the quality of our lives. If we can this do for the natural changes life brings, then we should do it even more in the sexual and communication departments.

This chapter aims to explore the quality of communication and sex. There is an expiration date on the member as well. In fact, it is not only the member in question, it is also the mind. When the mind is renewed, then the expiration date is renewed. When you have a refreshed mind, you have a fresh way of seeing, thinking, and treating one another. If you think you are old, then you will act old. If you try to keep yourself fresh and renewed in lovemaking and communication, the marriage will have great quality.

Too many couples are concerned about and proud of the number of years they have spent together—the *quantity* of the marriage. What I speak of is the *quality* of the marriage. Many couples know how to have quantity in their marriage, but their marriages lack quality. The sex is lacking. The communication is lacking. The passion is lacking, but they have the years. The sexual positions are the same. The communication is the same, and all the other things are the same, but they have the years.

This chapter challenges you to say, "I will strive for quality in my marriage. My marriage will get better and never stay the same!" Many things inhibit marriages in the bedroom, but boredom or lack of trying to make changes should not be present in the Christian bedroom. The more changes you make, the stronger the marriage will become. Again, it is not just quantity of years of marriage but quality that couples should strive for.

Life is nothing but trying to make your own life better. Making your life better does not come automatically. Something must be done to accomplish this. If we understand we have to do something to get something, then it is time for us to do the same thing in our marriages. We have to take action to keep the quality great. We have to take some action and take the love to another level.

The quantity and quality of the marriage is up to you because the expiration date is on your member. You must make changes to stop the expiration and renew your options. Change your hair, change your clothing, do something to create a change in the marriage. If you stay the same, then you get the same. Yet, if you turn the page and do something different, you will surely get something different and turn the page in your marriage.

Whatever it took to get the marriage, needs to be done to keep the marriage. If, in the beginning, you could not keep your hands off each other, you must begin again. Smart couples do not just keep each other; they relish each other in all avenues of the marriage.

Stop using age as an excuse. You may not feel sexy, wives, so buy sexy clothing to put you in the mood. Just to remind you: the clothes are coming off any way. Remember it is not the body, but you who decide whether you are sexy or not. Use or loose it, the choice is up to every couple.

IT IS NOT NASTY
(INSPIRED BY SONG OF SOLOMON)

IT IS NOT NASTY
(Inspired by Song of Solomon)

I have heard this adjective nasty applied to sex for many years. Sex is not nasty for married men and women. In fact, it is the closest thing to heaven on earth when a married man takes his time and examines every part of his wife's body. It is not nasty when he takes his fingers and starts from her toes and anoints every part of her body. It is not nasty when a husband locks the door and the music is on and he is about to enter her whispering eye when the kids are home. Oh, no that husband is not nasty, he's just loving. It is not nasty when the wife feels her husband touch and not his hands.

No, it is not nasty when he runs her bath and slowly and precisely rubs and rinses ever part of her body. He understands that the breast and vagina are wonderful, but he knows that those are the main course. Oh no, it is not nasty when a man discovers and touches all the erotic zones of his wife's body. Despite the children and marks to prove it, he still touches every part because he is a part of her.

Yes. He clears his schedule so he can spend time with her. When he can afford it, he takes her to a hotel and has hot passionate talk and sex with his wife to let her know it is not just her body, but also her mind that he loves.

For her part, a wife will tell her husband exactly what she desires. She will not hesitate to explain her body to him because she knows her body. She will explain the location of her love spots. She will explain where to kiss and how hard or soft to kiss.

Oh yes, she will tell him that yesterday she needed a teacher, but today she needs a beast in her bed. Yesterday she needed a doctor to examine her but tonight she needs a firefighter to deal with her fire. Oh no, it is not nasty, it is beautiful. Yesterday she needed a provider, but tonight she needs one to love and touch her all night long.

The only thing nasty is when a spouse gives his love and passion to another. Nasty is when a man redefines his vows to another man but continues his love affair with his wife. That is nasty.

However, when a husband loves his wife to the point that she yells and becomes his cheerleader that is not nasty. No, there is nothing nasty about that—it is a beautiful thing.

Faking orgasms is never an issue, because faking is the same as lying about spousal intentions. If I lie about an orgasm, I can lie about a phone number. If I lie about orgasms, I can lie about a late night call. I will not lie in or outside the bed; for a lie is an untruth and the only 'un' that I want in my marriage is undress.

It is a beautiful thing when men and women can walk past others and forsake others to come home to their respective mates. It is not nasty when a husband forsakes all others at work and church and in the neighborhood and brings his member home to his wife. No, it is not nasty when she greets him at the door with only a coat on after the kids are gone. No sir, that is not nasty. It is not nasty to wreck the hair and suit because you cannot keep your hands off each other.

It is not nasty when, after five, ten, twenty years, or more, a husband still gets engrossed in his member when he sees his wife with or without clothes. It is not nasty when the wife touches, he responds. It is not nasty when the husband wears something his wife cannot keep her hands off. No, it is not nasty.

No, it is not nasty when a wife shops at a sexy clothing store to let her husband see clothes that only have a wearing life of 20 seconds or minutes. Oh, no, it is not nasty when a wife and husband work out their PC muscles in order to last and squeeze every drop. It is not nasty to go to a sensual place and shop together for items to enhance the relationship. Not it is not nasty it is good.

No, it is not nasty when a man turns off his cell phone and TV to have close and intimate time with his wife. It is not nasty when he tells his boys or play station, "No," but he says, "Yes," to a girl flick his wife picked out. No, it is not nasty but wonderful when husband and wife can be naked and spoon the night away.

A wise wife would rather have a husband who is honest then a so-called perfect man who is dishonest. No, she is blessed with this man in her life. She loves this man. Therefore, because he loves and is faithful to her, she will mess up his world tonight. She has no doubt of his faithfulness.

It is not nasty when she turns to him 2 am in the morning and tells him your wish is my command. It is not nasty when she has issues on her mind and she allows a climax from her husband to be the eraser of pain. No, it is not nasty when she allows her husband to watch her slowly dress undress and dress again.

No, it is not nasty when she leaves a special package in his briefcase or in his lunch bag to remind him what is waiting for him at home.

No, it is not nasty for a husband to go buy the monthly needs for his wife. No, it is not nasty.

It is not nasty when the wife can make her husband feel good without him jumping the gun. She can play supermarket with him by touching, feeling, squeezing and smelling without him coming off the shelf until mommy says so. No, it is not nasty when the wife can do a strip search of her husband to the point that if she wants to arrest him he goes quietly and without incident.

No, it is not nasty when the wife says "I am your candy bar tonight because you been good to me."

No, it is not nasty when a wife sends a text message and after the husband reads it, he asks God for strength tonight to accomplish the entire bedroom request of his wife.

No, it is not nasty when a husband puts on nothing but his wife favorite cologne when he goes to bed. No, it is not nasty to experience the power of love and the union of one. No, it is not nasty in Eden.

No, it is not nasty when the wife becomes the director and actress and the husband becomes the stud in a sensual union during the night. No it is not nasty its heaven on earth.

No, it is not nasty when they wake in the arms of each other after a night of passion. No, it is not nasty when they cannot find each other under wears after the deed is done.

No, it is not nasty. It is not nasty when a wife finds her husband clean from the smell of another woman on his member. It is not nasty that when she kisses him with red lipstick in the morning its still red by the time he comes home.

It is not nasty for a husband to go underwear shopping for his wife. It is not nasty if for tonight, she is Wonder women and he is Superman. It is not nasty if he is Daredevil and she is Elektra.

It is not nasty if for a time they play Adam and Eve without the figs. No, it is not nasty that once the kids are gone they turn their home into the Garden of Eden.

It is not nasty if the husband prefers fishnet than regular cotton stockings. No, it is not nasty if she wears the heels and for that day she is taller than he.

In addition a wife says, "You are accountable and you are not down low; in fact you are up high because you decided to commit and become committed to me husband and I SHALL commit to you." A wife says, "What and how do you want it tonight? Because tonight I am Sarah and I call you lord." Oh, she loves you because there are no texts, phones, or dramas hindering the relationship.

The husband walks past the home wreckers, prostitutes, and came home without another woman's smell or body odor on him.

No, it is not nasty when she can check his phone and see no strange women on his index. It is beautiful how she checks and questions his credit cards and with every honest and truthful answer, he gives a smile.

No, it is beautiful when her husband ignites things in his wife to do the deed. It is not nasty that she touches him at 3:00 a.m., and he calls her name and not the name of a stranger. It is beautiful when he feels her, and she sings his name. It is wonderful when her husband touches and she does not pull away. Oh yeah, that is not nasty. It is wonderful.

It is wonderful when the wife rewards her husband for being the only man in the clothing store waiting patiently. It is wonderful when she turns, and he pays, and later, at home in the bedroom, she pays.

It is all give and take. In addition, after the babies, marks, and changes, the husband yet desires his wife—it is not just the external but also the internal he desires.

No, it is not nasty when she rewards him for never removing his wedding ring. Oh, she loves him because she can trust him. She knows when she smells him she smells herself. When she does the laundry, there are no phone numbers or condoms in his pants.

No, it is not nasty when between them their are no STDs. It is beautiful that in the twilight of their years, the wife can still do what the doctors cannot do—she can heal the pain with her touch.

No, it is not nasty when the child knocks on the door and the husband has to cover the wife because the child hears mommy calling out passionately. Oh, it is not nasty when it happens. When the husband cannot keeps his hands off his wife that is not nasty. After the years have gone by, the sizes have gone up, and they still desire one another. That is not nasty.

No, it is not nasty when the wife may be a missionary or play the 'mother' at church, but at home; she knows how to put a smile on her husband even before he gets home. She understands the power of a tinted car window and she touches her husband on the way from church to home. She has put a smile on his face because he is known as a faithful husband. He desires whatever she is going to give him today.

She is ready to cook up a love meal that is full of erotic

talk and love that keeps her husband wanting and coming back for more. Oh yes, in church she is devoutly religious, but at home she knows how to take care of her husband and her husband only. She knows how to entice and love him at the same time. It is not nasty when she is a lamb at church but a lioness to her husband at home.

Oh, no, it is not nasty, it is downright pleasing to God when a man roars and a wife chimes in after orgasms. No, it is not nasty when the man files his fingernails so when he touches her there are no sharp edges.

When He parts the waters and love and passion come forth, that is not nasty that is wonderful and beautiful in the eyes of God. No, husband and wife of the highest God, this is not nasty. It is called God's creation and gift.

It is Not Nasty. It is lovely.

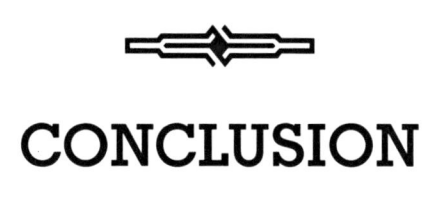

CONCLUSION

Conclusion

I pray this book has opened the eyes of many. The following are more scripture references toward sensual married sex between husband and wife (All Bible Verses uses New Living Translation:

Proverbs 5: 15 Drink water from your own well – share your love only with your wife.[F10] 16 Why spill the water of your springs in public, having sex with just anyone?[F11] 17 You should reserve it for yourselves. Don't share it with strangers. 18 Let your wife be a fountain of blessing for you. Rejoice in the wife of your youth. 19 She is a loving doe, a graceful deer. Let her breasts satisfy you always. May you always be captivated by her love. 20 Why be captivated, my son, with an immoral woman, or embrace the breasts of an adulterous woman? 21 For the LORD sees clearly what a man does, examining every path he takes. 22 An evil man is held captive by his own sins; they are ropes that catch and hold him. 23 He will die for lack of self-control; he will be lost because of his incredible folly.

Matthew 19: 4 Haven't you read the Scriptures? Jesus

replied. They record that from the beginning 'God made them male and female.' 5 And he said, 'This explains why a man leaves his father and mother and is joined to his wife, and the two are united into one.' 6 Since they are no longer two but one, let no one separate them, for God has joined them together. 7 Then why did Moses say a man could merely write an official letter of divorce and send her away? they asked. 8 Jesus replied, Moses permitted divorce as a concession to your hard-hearted wickedness, but it was not what God had originally intended. 9 And I tell you this, a man who divorces his wife and marries another commits adultery – unless his wife has been unfaithful. 10 Jesus' disciples then said to him, Then it is better not to marry! 11 Not everyone can accept this statement, Jesus said. Only those whom God helps. 12 Some are born as eunuchs, some have been made that way by others, and some choose not to marry for the sake of the Kingdom of Heaven. Let anyone who can, accept this statement.

1 Corinthians 7: 1 Now about the questions you asked in your letter. Yes, it is good to live a celibate life. 2 But because there is so much sexual immorality, each man should have his own wife, and each woman should have her own husband. 3 The husband should not deprive his wife of sexual intimacy, which is her right as a married woman, nor should the wife deprive her husband. 4 The wife gives authority over her body to her husband, and the husband also gives authority over his body to his wife. 5 So do not deprive each other of sexual relations. The only exception to this rule would be the agreement of both husband and wife to refrain from sexual intimacy for a limited time, so they can give themselves more completely to prayer. Afterward they should come together again so that Satan won't be able to tempt them because of their

lack of self-control. 6 This is only my suggestion. It is not meant to be an absolute rule. 7 I wish everyone could get along without marrying, just as I do. However, we are not all the same. God gives some the gift of marriage, and to others he gives the gift of singleness. 8 Now I say to those who aren't married and to widows – it's better to stay unmarried, just as I am. 9 But if they can't control themselves, they should go ahead and marry. It is better to marry than to burn with lust.

Hebrews 13:4 Give honor to marriage, and remain faithful to one another in marriage. God will surely judge people who are immoral and those who commit adultery.

Without a doubt, God needs to be in the center of your marriage. If you needed God at the altar during your wedding vows, how much more do you need him after the wedding is over?

Once you find God, **the author of sex**, put the book down and enjoy the gift God has given every husband and wife.